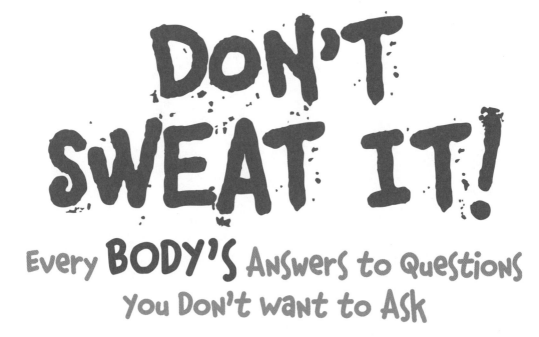

# DON'T SWEAT IT!

## Every BODY'S Answers to Questions You Don't want to Ask

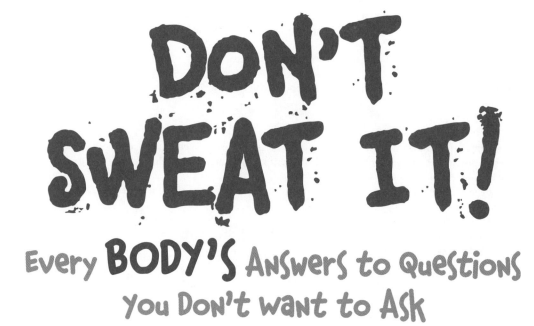

# DON'T SWEAT IT!

## Every BODY'S Answers to Questions You Don't want to Ask

### Marguerite Crump

Edited by Elizabeth Verdick

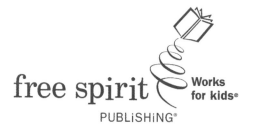

free spirit
PUBLISHING®

Works
for kids®

**Library of Congress Cataloging-in-Publication Data**
Crump, Marguerite, 1955–
Don't sweat it! : every body's answers to questions you don't want to ask : a guide for young people / Marguerite Crump.
   p. cm.
Includes bibliographical references and index.
Summary: An introduction to common concerns of adolescence, such as acne and body odor, covering the physical changes of puberty and offering tips on caring for oneself from head to toe.
ISBN 1-57542-114-3
1. Youth—Health and hygiene—Juvenile literature. 2. Adolescence—Juvenile literature. [1. Puberty. 2. Adolescence. 3. Health. 4. Cleanliness.] I. Title.

RJ140 .C784 2002
613'.0433—dc21
                                                                                    2002007021

Cover design by Marieka Heinlen
Interior book design by Crysten Puszczykowski
Illustrations by Chris Sharp
Index compiled by Randl Ockey

10 9 8 7 6 5 4 3 2 1
Printed in Canada

**Free Spirit Publishing Inc.**
217 Fifth Avenue North, Suite 200
Minneapolis, MN 55401-1299
(612) 338-2068
help4kids@freespirit.com
*www.freespirit.com*

The following are registered trademarks of Free Spirit Publishing Inc.:
FREE SPIRIT®
FREE SPIRIT PUBLISHING®
SELF-HELP FOR TEENS®
SELF-HELP FOR KIDS®
WORKS FOR KIDS®
THE FREE SPIRITED CLASSROOM®

free spirit
PUBLISHING®
Works for kids®

# DEDICATION

To my wonderful parents, who gave me the freedom and encouragement to find my own way—however far off the beaten path. — M.K.C.

# ACKNOWLEDGMENTS

This book was made possible with help from many teachers, parents, and students, who provided hilarious and insightful information and comments. Thanks to my husband and friends for their support, and thanks to Free Spirit Publishing for making this book possible.

# Contents

# INTRODUCTION

Lately, you may have noticed body changes happening around you and inside you. If so, you're probably somewhere between the ages of nine and thirteen—maybe older. During these years, change is the name of the game. You begin to look, act, and most of all feel different. Even if you haven't noticed many changes in yourself, you've probably seen some in your friends.

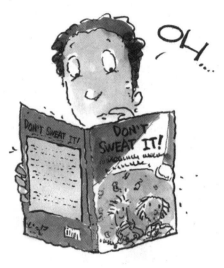

What are these changes all about? *Puberty*—the time when your body begins the passage from childhood to adulthood. But this isn't a book on puberty. It's a book on how to take the "P.U." out of puberty.

As you know, many of the physical changes you're dealing with now (or will be soon) aren't the stuff of polite conversation: sweaty armpits, stinky feet, and bad breath, to name a few. That's just for starters: You'll also experience changes in your genitals—those parts down below— changes you'd probably like to know more about, if only you weren't afraid to ask. After all, how often do you hear people openly discussing pubic hair? Or body odor? How about bathroom habits? Sweat glands? Oily hair? Head lice? Toe jam? Not often. These things are embarrassing! They're *private*. But they're part of life.

This book discusses the often unmentionable changes and personal health issues that are hard to talk about face-to-face. In the privacy of this book, you'll learn all about good hygiene—why it's important, how it helps, and how to stay clean every day.

I never set out to learn so much about the human body and how it works. But in my job as a health educator, I was asked to consult with school nurses about the health topic they most needed to present to their students. The nurses and students wanted more information on personal hygiene—something people deal with daily but don't talk much about. The more I learned, the more I shared with students through workshops and presentations.

I realized that sensitive topics can be a lot of fun. Students laughed when I talked about dandruff, armpit hair, toenail care, and food caught in your teeth. When these topics were discussed in a group setting, they no longer seemed as uncomfortable or embarrassing.

That's why I decided to write this book—to help kids like you understand that body changes are normal for everyone, and so are the feelings that go with them. You may feel up, down, or somewhere in between at any given time on any given day. Being worried, excited, uncomfortable, or "weirded out" is all part of puberty and growing up.

What helps? Knowing yourself and taking care of yourself. Feeling good is up to you—and this book will tell you how.

## ABOUT THIS BOOK

You're about to learn how to take excellent care of yourself from head to toe. Here's what you'll find:

### 1. HAIR: Crowning Glory or Constant Struggle?

Discover why hair seems to have a mind of its own and how you can better care for yours.

### 2. FACE Facts

Learn why skin—your body's largest organ—needs special attention, especially on your face.

### 3. Your MOUTH (An Amusement Park for Germs)

Find out why germs love your mouth and how you can make it a cleaner, healthier place.

### 4. Helping HANDS

Understand why your hands can be your first defense against germs and illness, *if* you wash them once in a while.

### 5. BODY ODOR BaSicS

Get the inside scoop on sweating and body odor—
and find out how to keep B.O. at bay.

### 6. Those PARTS BELOW

Learn about your private parts (genitals) and why
what's happening down there is such a big hairy deal.

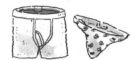

### 7. Sweet FEET

Take a look at how to keep your feet as fresh and
clean as possible, even if you play sports.

Throughout this book, you'll read lots of fascinating facts and myths about the human body (some will even surprise you). Along the way, you just might realize that your body is an *amazing* machine. Taking good care of it now—and always—will help keep it in top form.

If you want to write to me, I'd love to hear from you. You can reach me here:

Marguerite Crump
c/o Free Spirit Publishing
217 Fifth Avenue North, Suite 200
Minneapolis, MN 55401-1299
Email: help4kids@freespirit.com

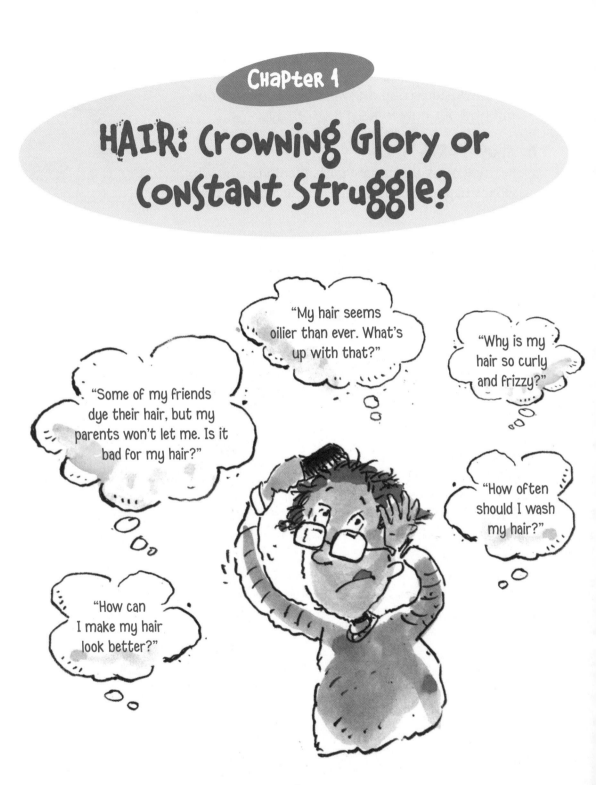

Have you ever been on a quick errand and unexpectedly run into some girl or boy you wanted to impress? There you are in the middle of Bargains Galore, trying to make witty small talk while all you can think is, "What's my hair doing right now?" The first thing you do when you're back in the car is flip down the mirror and check yourself out. Yikes! Your hair's doing some goofy-looking backbend, and you feel like a dork. Before you vow to never leave home without first spending an hour in front of the mirror, remember that *everyone* has hair anxiety at times.

Hair can definitely make you feel stressed. It's the first thing you notice when you look in the mirror—and let's face it, you check out everyone else's hair, too. Does this mean you're shallow? Surely not. Hair just happens to be a noticeable feature. You can't help but see it first.

## HAIR AWARENESS

Remember those carefree little-kid days when you hopped out of bed, threw on some clothes, and headed out to play without giving your hair a second thought? You may have run a comb through it at the urging of your mom or dad, but your hair wasn't a high priority. Your parents probably made your haircut appointments or cut your hair for you. Those days are gone. If you're like most people your age, you now have Good Hair Days or Bad Hair Days. You may freak out about frizzies, curse your stick-straight locks, regret that new buzz cut, or spend countless hours trying new hair products and styles.

Hair's a big deal—and it's been that way through history. As long as there have been people on Earth, there have been signs that they paid attention to their hair. Even primitive cave people used feathers and bones to keep their hair out of their way and to show their social status.

By looking at artifacts (such as combs, hairpins, paintings, and poetry), archeologists have found that Ancient Egyptians were some of the earliest people to place importance on the beauty of their hair. While the Egyptians loved long locks fixed in fancy styles, the hot and dusty climate made long hair not only hot but also a happy home for bugs. That's why the people favored cropped hair and shaved heads, and added on hair extensions or dyed wigs.

## Fact!

Throughout history, people have worn their hair in styles that follow their religious beliefs. Christian and Buddhist monks shaved their heads to show they gave up worrying about vain things like their hair. Muslim men left one long lock of hair on their shaved heads, believing Allah would use it to pull them into heaven.

★

"Dreadlocks" are long, matted rolls of hair, woven loosely together. Jamaican people with this hairstyle were considered rebels the police "dreaded" seeing. Today, people from all different countries and races wear their hair in "dreads."

In fact, wigs have long been a traditional fashion statement—whether the gray wig of a British barrister (lawyer) or the black, lacquered wig of a Japanese geisha. People today still wear wigs or may get hair extensions to give the appearance of longer, thicker hair.

You may pay a lot more attention to your hair these days, but have you ever really *thought about* your hair? Your scalp is like a factory, working day and night to grow the hair you know and love or love to hate. Your hair is made up of *keratin,* a thin, colorless substance that also makes up your nails. There are three basic layers of hair: the *cuticle* (the thin, colorless outside layer that protects the hair), the *cortex* (the middle part that gives hair strength and determines its color and texture), and the *medulla* (the hair's soft center).

The hair root sits beneath the skin surface in a hair *follicle,* which looks like a tiny pit; blood vessels flow into the area and help the hair grow. All that stuff you wash and comb is actually dead. While commercials may make you think you've got to feed the "thirsty" hair on your head, your hair isn't waiting around like some sweaty athlete needing a water bottle. The only actual live tissue in your hair is in the root. The parts you deal with every day are thousands of hair shafts.

All those hairs on your head are on different time schedules, growing and falling out depending on what phase they're in. They start out in a heavy-growth phase; next, they take a little rest. Then it's out with the old and in with the new, as fresh hairs push their way through. It's a good thing those hairs are on different schedules—you wouldn't want them all to be in the resting stage at once, or you'd be wading through hair in your bathtub and there'd be nothing to comb when you looked in the mirror.

While it's a bit hard to count all the hairs on a human head, scientists say there are between 60,000–150,000. If you took a wet wad of tissue and wiped it around the bathroom floor, you'd be shocked at how much of your family's hair is there. That is, unless cleaning the bathroom is one of your regular chores—in which case, you're well aware of how much hair lands on the floor.

Have you ever reached down to clear out a slow bathroom drain and come up with a huge, goopy clump of hair? Disgusting! (It *is* a bit curious that we find hair so appealing when it's artfully arranged on someone's head, but once it's off the head we recoil in horror.) No, this isn't a sign that everyone in your family is going bald. They're probably shedding about 50–150 hairs every day, which is normal.

When you're a kid, your hair is at a fuller volume than at any other time in your life. It's also shiny and

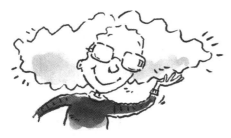

healthy looking because the oil glands are working at a good pace. And your hair color is brighter—it hasn't yet begun to darken, which it may do when you're in your teens or twenties.

During the teen years, hair gets oilier because the oil glands start working overtime, secreting *sebum,* or skin oil, into the follicle. Sebum moistens your scalp and makes your hair shiny—but it can also turn your hair into Grease City. Those tiny oil glands can make a big mess on your scalp during puberty.

Want to find out if your hair is healthy? Try this: Grasp one of your hairs when it's wet and give it a slow, gentle pull. It should stretch quite a bit before it finally breaks. Healthy hair can be stretched to about 25 percent of its length without breaking. Believe it or not, a healthy hair is stronger than a steel wire of the same size. If your

---

## Fact!

Hair grows at different rates, depending on many factors. It grows faster in warm weather than in cold weather, faster in the morning than in the afternoon, and slowest at night.

★

Human hair is used as an additive to some foods. What's that you say? We eat hair on purpose!? An amino acid called L-cysteine can be made from human hair and is added to foods like bread, pizza dough, and some kinds of snacks. The hair mostly comes from China and is processed in chemical plants to convert it to a powder. You may not be able to see this additive listed in a product's ingredients because the label might say "dough enhancer" or "natural flavoring."

**Fact!**

The color of your hair influences how many hairs you have on your head. If you're a redhead, you have about 80,000 hairs. Brunettes have around 100,000 hairs, and blonds have about 120,000 hairs. How can this be? Blonds have more hairs on their heads because their hair tends to be thinner than darker varieties. No one knows why.

⭐

There's no such thing as gray hair. When melanin stops producing color in hair, the hair becomes white. If you look closely at a grandparent's head, you'll see that what you thought were gray hairs are white hairs alongside hair that still has color.

hair doesn't have elasticity (it breaks easily when stretched), it may be damaged from chlorine, sun, a perm, dyes, or heat from a hair dryer or curling iron.

## Your Hair Color

If you look around your classroom or even at the family members around your dinner table, you'll see a wide variety of hair colors. Hair is usually categorized as black, blond, red, or brown, but some heads of hair are pretty hard to describe. Reddish blond? Blondish red? Blackish brown? Dirty blond? Jet black? Whatever your color, it's unique like you are.

The color is determined by *melanin,* which is present in your pigment, or coloring, cells. (Melanin also makes your skin have a dark color or freckles.) The more melanin you have in your hair, the darker it will be. When you get old someday and your pigment cells stop working, your hair will turn white.

## Curly or Straight?

The shape of your hair follicles, or those little pits in your scalp that hold your hair roots, determines your hair type. So if your follicles have a circular shape, you get straight hair. Oval follicles mean curly hair. Flat, curved follicles produce hair 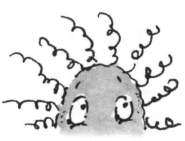 that's tightly curled or kinky. There are also chemical bonds in hair that create a curly or straight look. If you get a perm or relax your hair, you're breaking down those chemical bonds.

Have you ever looked in the mirror and wished you could change your hair from straight to curly, or vice versa? It's normal to want the exact opposite of what you were born with. Suppose you want your hair to straighten out, but its natural curl makes it bounce into corkscrew shapes. Or you'd like wavy, full hair, but it just lies as flat as a sheet of paper. Your hair type was decided long before you were born, thanks to your parents. If you had a nickel for every person throughout time who's tried to force their hair into doing what it doesn't want to do, you'd be rolling in millions!

Whether your hair is dark or light, curly or straight, it's yours. And it's up to you to take good care of it. The more you care for your hair, the better it will look—no matter what type of hair you were born with. Besides, there's a hair product for just about every situation.

## BASIC HAIR CARE

Think about your morning hair routine. Do you wash your hair, run your fingers through it, and head out the door? Or do you allow an extra hour for all that washing, conditioning, drying, styling, and spraying? (It's exhausting just thinking about it.)

If you spend a lot of time fussing with your hair in the morning and checking yourself in the mirror all day long, you might need some tips on keeping it simple. On the other hand, if your idea of hair care is licking your palm and slicking down your bangs, you could use some tips on keeping it clean. Either way, you've come to the right place.

### washing and Conditioning

You only have to look in the hair-care aisle of any drugstore to see that you can buy a lot of stuff for your hair. But do you really need so many products? Couldn't you just grab a bar of soap and use it on your hair, too? There's nothing wrong with doing that if you're already soaking

Fact!

Forensic scientists—or super sleuths who help solve crimes—can study one hair left at a crime scene to figure out its owner's sex, age, and race.

"I don't like my hair one bit. My mom has curly hair, and my dad has straight hair so my hair is straight except for one curl that sticks out. I look like a dork."
—Sarah, 12

wet in a shower and there's no shampoo in sight, but soap isn't good for your hair. It will dry it out and leave a dull film. Shampoos have special detergents designed to make a foamy lather that will leave your hair clean, healthy, and shiny.

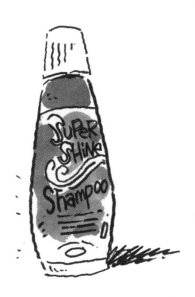

There are so many shampoos available that it's hard to know which one to choose. And who could possibly understand all those big words in the lists of ingredients on shampoo bottles? Your best bet is to figure out whether your hair type is dry, oily, or normal. Then pick a cleansing or conditioning shampoo—whichever kind suits you. Cleansing shampoos for all different hair types are supposed to remove the oil and dirt from hair. Conditioning shampoos clean and condition hair, making it softer, thicker, and easier to style. If you use a conditioning shampoo, you don't have to use a separate conditioner after washing. To confuse matters, there are also moisturizing shampoos—which are conditioning shampoos that "lock in" moisture.

Hair conditioners are products that contain ingredients to "coat" your hair and smooth it out. Conditioners can make your hair look fuller and keep it from getting charged up with static electricity. You also can find "deep" conditioners or "intensive" conditioners that you leave on your hair for a period of time to seal in even more moisture.

If you have oily hair, wash it daily with a cleansing shampoo designed to cut through oil and dirt. You can use a light conditioner on your hair as often as needed (every other day or so). If you have normal hair, choose a cleansing or conditioning shampoo that's designed for your hair type; use a light conditioner, if you'd like. If you're on an athletic team or if you often exercise outdoors, your hair may get sweaty and dirty. Feel free to wash it more often.

For dry, frizzy, or coarse hair, try a moisturizing or conditioning shampoo. You also can look for "low Ph" or "Ph-balanced" shampoos, which won't strip away oil (you need the oil to lubricate your dry hair). To keep the oils in, wash your hair only a few times per week. Always follow up with a conditioner; use a deep or intensive conditioner every so often, too.

People of African-American heritage have hair that requires gentle, less-frequent handling with shampoos, especially if it's been straightened with relaxers or curling irons (these processes weaken hair). You can look for shampoos and conditioners that are designed for your hair type. If you're active in sports and want to remove sweat from your hair, try rinsing it out instead of shampooing too often, which will strip away oils.

No matter what your hair type, you've probably heard of "Lather. Rinse. Repeat." If not, go check out the directions on the nearest shampoo bottle. Some brilliant shampoo-maker of the past must have thought this would be a great way to sell more shampoo (because the more you use, the more you buy). By all means, lather and rinse, but it's not necessary to repeat. If your hair type is dry, shampooing it twice will remove too many oils. Even if your hair is oily, lathering up twice isn't needed. Save yourself some time and money by ignoring that old rule.

If you don't have much spare cash, you may be using whatever shampoo and conditioner your family has. That's okay, too, because most shampoos work fine on most hair. TV commercials may lead you to believe that shampoos and conditioners are highly scientific and you *must* have the right formula for your particular hair. The most important thing is to simply keep your hair clean.

Expensive doesn't always mean better. There are plenty of low-cost shampoos that work as well as the ones at fancy salons. Just because some people buy the expensive stuff doesn't mean their hair will be any cleaner or softer than yours. If you buy hair products with your own money, you can shop smart by choosing a conditioning shampoo instead of two separate products.

Fact!

The foods you eat can affect your hair. Foods that are good for your hair include eggs, meat, cheese, seeds and nuts, carrots, green vegetables, citrus fruits, milk, and fish.

## Combing, Brushing, and Styling

Are you one of those people who shows up at school with the hairstyle that Mother Nature gave you overnight, otherwise known as Bed Head? If so, ask yourself this: When was the last time you thought your hair looked fabulous after falling asleep on the bus, much less after a whole night with your hair scrunched into a pillow?

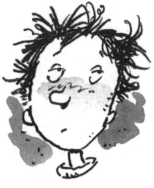

It's time to take out that comb or brush, and use it every day. (True, there are trendy hairstyles that mimic Bed Head, but even *they* take work to achieve.) It's best to put a little effort into your hair routine. Why not start today?

Maybe you're the other extreme. Are your two best friends your hairbrush and hair dryer? Try not to spend too much time with these styling tools, because your hair doesn't need that kind of wear and tear. For best results, gently towel dry your hair a bit, wet comb it with a wide-toothed comb, and then begin styling with a brush and hairdryer if needed. (Look for soft, flexible hairbrushes. Natural bristle brushes are easiest on your hair; soft synthetic brushes with rounded tips are good options, too.) Use a medium heat setting on your dryer, instead of going for the inferno level. Dry until your hair is only a little damp, so it's not gasping for moisture afterward. Keep that dryer moving and don't blast your hair in one spot for too long.

Be sure to keep your hairbrush clean. Have you ever looked closely at one of those things? Behold the dense mat of tangled hairs. Granted, they're *your* hairs, but you really should give that nest a good cleaning. Take a slender tool like a screwdriver or pencil and slide it under the hair to lift it off the brush. Soak the brush in warm water with a bit of shampoo to remove oil and dirt. Then rinse the brush in clean water and let it dry face down on a towel. Combs need a good soaking and scrubbing every so often, too.

At your age, you may be playing around with different styles for your hair. Your hair is probably strong enough to withstand all the experimenting. This is the fun part, because you get to be an artist with your hair. Here's a rundown of some of the many products you can use to make your hair heed your command:

* **BALMS:** tame the frizzies in curly hair and add shine. Use a dab of this on your wet hair, then style.

* **GELS:** give shape and shine to all hair types. They can be applied to wet hair for a wet look, or they can be used on wet hair to help shape it as it dries.

* **HAIRSPRAY:** holds hair in a certain style. The aerosol sprays dry fast and cover a large area quickly. Spritz sprays are wetter. Look for the holding strength your hair needs.

* **MOLDING MUD:** holds curls or spikes in hair and can give a wet look.

* **MOUSSE:** adds volume to thin, fine hair.

* **POMADES:** smooth out curly hair.

* **VOLUMIZERS:** make thin hair look thicker. Use on wet hair before styling.

To save money, look for these products at discount stores. Keep the receipt so you can exchange any product you're not happy with.

# DON'T TRY THIS AT HOME

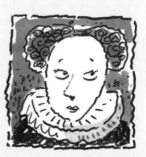

If you've ever questioned how people are willing to do anything because it's the trend of the moment, you only have to look at a painting of a woman from the Middle Ages. Ever see those ladies with the super high foreheads? They plucked their hairline back several inches to make their forehead seem higher. Ouch!

In the 1770s, wealthy women in Europe wore their hair built up over wire cages and powdered with starch to make it stand up to three feet high. They decorated these hairdos with feathers, ribbons, and jewels—as well as an occasional ornamental bird. These styles took hours to create, so they were left undisturbed for several weeks. Sometimes bugs moved into those "beehives."

## Haircuts and Perms

Styling aids are fun, but the best thing you can do is start with a *good* haircut—from a salon or barber shop. You may think you can trim your own hair (or your mom or dad may offer to do it), but hair cutting is best left to experts. Home haircuts often turn out badly, especially when people use dull scissors they found in their junk drawers.

That's not to say that everyone has lots of money to spend on fancy haircuts. You don't have to go to the top salon in town. Bargain hair-cutting salons and walk-in places are good options; so are beauty schools. Barber shops are inexpensive, too. Boys head to the barber shop more often than girls do, but girls can go to one for a simple cut or bang trim. Barbers have mastered short haircuts and can usually do the job quickly. The best way to scout out a good hairstylist or barber is to ask friends, neighbors, and relatives for any suggestions. Try to get your hair cut every six weeks to two months.

Keep in mind that *you* are the customer, and you deserve great service. Don't be shy about telling the barber or stylist what you want done. You've got to speak up before they start in with the scissors. You can ask for their opinion about what would work best for you; even better, bring along a photo of someone who's got the style you want. Unless you like to take big risks, don't say, "Oh, just be creative"—especially if the stylist has scary hair. Be specific and you're more likely to get what you want.

What if you end up with a lousy haircut anyway? Ask a parent to go with you to talk to the stylist or manager, so you can get the cut fixed or get your money back. Even the shortest haircuts—painful as they may be—grow out eventually. (Hair grows an average of one half inch per month, in case you're wondering.) If people tease you, try not to let it get you down.

If your sister, brother, or best friend is the one who got a really bad haircut, whatever you do don't laugh. And don't make a crack like, "WHAT did you DO to your HAIR?" If your friend likes his or her new hairstyle, be supportive. After all, you might need someone's support if you decide to do something daring with your own appearance.

Salons offer other styling options, like perming, straightening, and coloring. Perms are designed to add curl to the hair; the opposite is straightening or relaxing the curl from hair. Both boys and girls can have these chemical processes done. If you're black, your hair may be naturally kinky or curly, and you may use relaxers and pressing combs to straighten it. To keep it from breaking and splitting, treat your hair with "greasy" products like deep conditioners and hot oil treatments. Use natural bristle hairbrushes and wide-toothed combs.

If you ever want to go straight or curly, it's nice to have these options, but don't overdo it—or the ends of your hair may start looking as dry and fuzzy as cotton candy. The important thing is to keep your hair healthy and find a style you love.

## Fact!

Most human hair stops growing when it's about 3 feet long, but some people have amazing hair-growing ability. In 1989 a woman in India was discovered to have hair 21 feet long—the longest recorded in the world.

✱

The permanent wave (perm) was invented by German Charles Nestle in 1906. He used a machine that had metal curlers hooked up to a source of electricity. Customers sat under the machine for 12 hours!

## Changing Your Hair Color

Today, teens are the fastest growing hair-coloring market. Whether you're thinking of going darker, lighter, hot pink, or lime green, a new hair color can make a statement about you. There are different methods for changing your color, and you can do it at home or a salon. *Temporary rinses* last only until you wash your hair. *Semi-permanent dyes* stay on through a number of washings but can only deposit a darker color on your hair (not lighten it). *Permanent dyes* don't wash out, but as new hairs grow in they'll be your original color.

If you decide to change your color, run the idea by your dad or mom before you take the plunge. By the way, you wouldn't be the first person to get the hot idea to let your best friend color your hair for you. Chances are, you might end up with fried hair in some never-before-seen shade. Before you try this, give some thought to how you'd feel if you walked into the school cafeteria with your new "do" and everyone couldn't stop staring. (Otherwise known as "hair don't.")

## COLOR KNOW-HOW

★ Choose a hair color close to your original color if you're going for a natural look.

★ If you realize you've made a mistake, get a hairdresser's help.

★ Use shampoos and conditioners specially designed for colored hair.

★ If your hair is really dry or damaged, hold off on the coloring so it doesn't get more fried.

★ Don't perm or relax your hair the day you color it, or you could dry it out more.

★ Wear a hat if you're in the sun—the sun's ultraviolet rays change the chemicals in hair color and can cause it to fade.

✱ If you spend time swimming in chlorinated pools, your best bet is to get a swim cap. Chlorine is a chemical salt that dries and weakens hair; chlorine also reacts with the chemicals in your hair if it's been colored, permed, or straightened. It's true that chlorine can turn blond hair green, so beware.

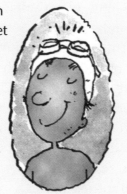

## HAIR PROBLEMS

It's spring, you're wearing a cool black T-shirt, and you suddenly realize there are snowflakes all over your shoulders. What's going on? *Dandruff.* There's a type of yeast on everyone's scalp, and this yeast feeds on the bacteria that's present in the oil on your head. (Nice, huh?) Some people are very sensitive to the yeast, and it starts to grow like crazy, producing those little white flakes.

Dandruff is itchy and uncomfortable, but it doesn't mean you have to hide your head in the sand like an ostrich. You can buy dandruff shampoo at any drugstore. If your dandruff is really bad (look for a pink scalp and greasy, yellow flakes), see a doctor as soon as you can.

What else makes your head itchy and uncomfortable? Good old head lice. They're the teeny, tiny critters that love to suck the blood on your scalp. Most people think this problem only happens to really young kids, but head lice aren't picky about age. Any head will do. You can't catch these bugs from an animal or from being outdoors—but you can catch them from your best friend. Head lice are passed from person to person. The number-one clue that you might have a problem is an itchy head. Have a parent or a school nurse check your

---

*Fact!*

In the 1800s, men began to darken their mustaches with dye. The first real hair color formula was created in 1825. Called Grecian Water, it was made of silver nitrate, water, and gum water. It was very popular—until people discovered that after using it repeatedly, it turned their hair purple.

✱

Archeologists have found head lice dried on mummies' heads, which means the insects have survived thousands of years of human attempts to get rid of them.

head under a strong light, using a magnifying glass. Look for the bugs and for tiny eggs stuck on hair shafts close to the scalp.

These little overnight guests won't leave unless you force them to. One way to get rid of lice is to try to smother them with olive oil. Lice-killing shampoos are available, too. Once you treat the hair, you have to comb out all the nits (babies) with a special nit comb. Lice can live for up to two days away from your head, so they may be hanging around in caps, pillows, sheets, towels, and other places your head has touched. If you get head lice, you'll have to wash clothing and bedding, and vacuum the furniture. The best prevention is to keep your stuff separate from other people's stuff at school or sports practice—and never share brushes and combs.

One thing to remember: an itchy scalp doesn't automatically mean dandruff or head lice. You may just have dry skin on your scalp, especially during winter when the air is drier. Or maybe you've been using lots of products (deep conditioners, dyes, gels, hairsprays) that have built up on your hair. Wash your hair as usual, but skip the additional products for a few days if needed. Your scalp may feel better.

## HAIR, HAIR EVERYWHERE

Everyone has one-of-a-kind hair. You may already have a style that works for you—and that's great if you do. Remember, though, that some kids may not have an awesome style, or can't quite figure out what to do with their "do." Be respectful of other people's style, even if it's no style.

What if *you* are the one getting teased or criticized about your hair? You're at a stage in your life when looks become more important. Some people you know may even seem to obsess about appearances and act like it's their mission in life to make nasty comments about others. They may act superior, but they're not. It's hard to ignore this behavior, but try to anyway. Don't take it too much to heart.

Keep experimenting—you'll eventually find a look that's right for you. The key is good hair care and working with what you've got. In other words, if you have straight black hair, don't try to make yourself into a curly-headed blond. If you've got a head of curls, why fight them? Who needs all that constant maintenance? You've got more important things to do.

# CHAPTER 2

# FACE Facts

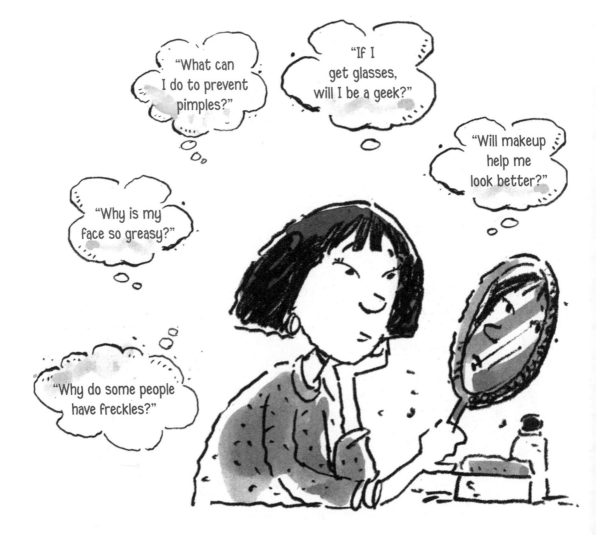

"What can I do to prevent pimples?"

"If I get glasses, will I be a geek?"

"Will makeup help me look better?"

"Why is my face so greasy?"

"Why do some people have freckles?"

**F**ace it: Your face says something about you. Do you want it to say that you're (A) healthy, confident, and nice to be around, or (B) a total slob? If you chose A, keep reading so you can learn lots of facts about taking good care of your fabulous face. If you picked B, you need help. This chapter may convince you that the face you show the world is worth taking care of.

## THE SKINNY ON YOUR SKIN

Does it seem as if you've got the world's largest oil slick on your face, or a big volcano is about to erupt on your nose? It's not time to call in the eco-disaster experts. You've probably got a case of oily skin or a big zit, like lots of people your age. Your skin is facing puberty, the time when you start growing into an adult.

Before and during puberty, the *hormones* in your body go a little wild. (Read more about those zinging hormones in Chapter 5, "Body Odor Basics" and Chapter 6, "Those Parts Below.") During this time of your life, your face changes along with the rest of your body.

Have you noticed that your facial features are growing and shifting? Is your nose bigger? How about your ears? Those parts that stick out might now stick out more than usual. Your eyebrows may get darker or bushier. And speaking of hair, you may have noticed more of that on your upper lip or chin, whether you're a boy or a girl. All of these changes are normal at this stage of life. So are skin changes—even the ones you may not be happy about.

It will take a few years for your skin to settle down. If that seems like forever, keep in mind that your skin will have its good days and bad days, just like your hair. (Read more about hair in Chapter 1, "Hair: Crowning Glory or Constant Struggle?") You can help keep your skin cleaner and clearer. A little skin care goes a long way.

If you're frustrated about your skin, try to look on the bright side. Consider what this miraculous organ does. For starters, skin keeps your insides in so your other organs aren't falling all over the floor. And skin keeps the outside out so water doesn't fill up your body each time it rains.

"I like my skin because it is white and black mixed."
—Takoreah, 9

Your skin repels water but has pores (tiny openings) that let out the sweat. That means your skin helps cool you off. Your skin repairs itself when you get a cut or scrape, and is home to the nerve endings that warn you if you touch something too hot. Maybe you thought all your skin did was break out the day of your big oral report?

There's more to your skin than what you see on the outside. Think back to when you slid into second base or fell while hiking—you probably got a red, angry-looking scrape. If you were to look closely at that wound, you might see several different layers. The top layer is known as the *epidermis,* or the layer that water can't penetrate. The *dermis* layer, in the middle, supports and shapes the epidermis. Your sweat glands, oil glands, blood vessels, hair roots, and nerves make their home in the dermis. The *subcutaneous* layer lies deep beneath and is mostly made up of fat. It acts as a cushion for your organs and helps keep you warm.

On average, your skin is only about one-sixteenth of an inch thick. That's about the size of a ballpoint pen tip. Now you can impress your science teacher with your vast knowledge of skin layers!

## Your Skin Coloring

Your skin color is unique, just like all of your other features and qualities. You may have skin that's darker or lighter than your friends'. Why are there so many different colors of skin? Because of *melanin,* or skin pigment. The melanin in skin cells helps determine the skin's color.

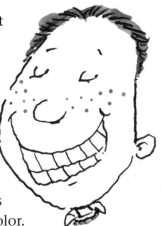

Darker-skinned people generally have more melanin, and it's more densely packed in their skin cells.

Whether you have dark or light skin, you may have freckles. These little dots of color tend to be more common among people who have light hair and fair skin. Some people are self-conscious about their freckles; others are proud of them.

Freckles appear as a result of time spent in the sun, which is why there are more of them on the face, hands, and legs—the parts of the body that get more sun exposure. If you're not a freckle lover, be sure to wear sunscreen (read more about that on pages 34–35) and be careful about how much time you spend in the sun. Even if you love your freckles, sunscreen is a must!

Maybe you've seen ads for fade creams and you wonder if you should use these products to make your freckles disappear. Fade creams usually are a waste of time and money because freckles are permanent. If you have big bucks to spend on freckle removal, a dermatologist (skin doctor) could someday freeze off your freckles, get rid of them using acids or an electric needle, or sand them off like rough spots on plywood. These methods are pretty drastic and could leave you with white spots or scars where the freckles used to be. So, maybe those freckles sound pretty good after all?

Other colorations on the skin include moles. These are spots where the pigment cells have done some serious growing. Moles can appear nearly anywhere on the body. Moles that appear on the face may be referred to as "beauty marks." These marks can be tan, brown, or black, and may be flat or slightly raised.

You may have moles that you don't think of as beautiful. In fact, you might be worried about how they look or whether people will tease you. Remind yourself that plenty of celebrities and models have moles or beauty

Fact!

The Crayola crayon company changed the color named Flesh to Peach in 1962 to recognize that people have skin of different colors. The company changed the color Indian Red to Chestnut in 1999 because some teachers thought kids wrongly assumed the color was supposed to represent Native-American skin color. Indian Red was actually named after a pigment found in India.

"I have a beauty mark. It doesn't bother me. It may bother some other people."
—Jessica, 10

marks that haven't slowed down their careers. If you're self-conscious about a mole, talk to a doctor about whether it can be removed safely.

Like moles, birthmarks can be a sensitive issue. These typically red or brown markings are present when you're born and are permanent. Many birthmarks are nests of pigment cells. Marks called *port-wine stains* form when lots of tiny blood vessels bunch together. Port-wine stains are usually red or purple, and they're often found on a person's neck or scalp.

If you've got a birthmark, you may feel that it's no big deal. On the other hand, you may be upset about it, especially if you and your friends are starting to focus more on appearances. Concealer sticks (a kind of makeup) are an option. Or you could talk to a doctor about laser-removal treatments.

## Your Skin Glands

The sebaceous glands live in the middle layer of your skin. They're like little factories for sebum, or skin oil. The sebaceous glands are mostly on your face and forehead, as well as on your scalp. When you hit puberty and your hormones start dancing around inside you, the sebaceous glands begin to produce more oil. More oil can mean more skin problems, which is why washing your face is important.

Your sebaceous glands have neighbors: your *sweat glands*. These little moisture-producers constantly receive messages from your nervous system. The messages tell the glands how much sweat to deliver to the skin's surface. The sweat is supposed to moisten your skin and cool you off. If your pores get clogged with oil and dirt, the sweat glands can't do their job very well—another good reason to wash up.

## What's Bacteria Got to Do with It?

You're surrounded by bacteria. They're in the air. They're on the surfaces you touch. They're outside and inside of your body. Bacteria are directly involved in everything from acne to stinky feet. When you think about it, though, bacteria aren't all bad. They actually help make our world possible.

Like the rest of us, bacteria have to eat. The difference is bacteria eat just about anything, including waste products and dead stuff. For example, if a dead fly hits the ground, bacteria eat the bug as it rots into the soil. Sounds gross, but without bacteria, we'd be knee-deep in dead stuff.

As human beings, we need bacteria in and on our bodies. In fact, most bacteria *help* more than harm. Some bacteria live inside the body and fight off organisms that don't belong there. Other kinds of bacteria live on the skin and eat away at the sebum.

Most people think of bacteria as those little organisms that make people sick. Some bacteria, like the kind found in raw meat or in *feces* (poop), can cause illness. That's why it's so important to wash your hands throughout the day (more on that in Chapter 4, "Helping Hands"). A good hand-washing gets rid of the "bad" bacteria that cause germs.

It's also important to keep the rest of your skin clean and free of bacteria. Your skin will feel fresher and look better if you tend to it each day. The good news is that skin care is easy once you know the basics.

## Caring for Your Skin

Now that you know how your suit of skin is designed, you can learn how to take care of it. You've probably heard that what you do to your skin today will show up tomorrow

**Fact!**

There are more than 2 million bacteria making their home on your chin, cheeks, and nose.

★

If all the liquid were removed from your body, about 10 percent of your dry body weight would be bacteria.

and years from now. That's no lie. You can choose the route that eventually leads to wrinkly, blotchy, saggy skin, or the one where your skin looks healthy even when you're old.

Of course, your genes play a role here, too. The color and appearance of your skin depends on what your parents and grandparents passed down to you. Whether they had clear skin or skin problems, there's a good chance you will, too. How you care for the skin you've been given makes a difference, though.

If you think skin care is only for girls, think again. In case you haven't noticed, wrinkles and sags don't look too great on men, either. If you're a boy, *acne* can happen to you just as easily as it can to a girl. (You can read more about acne on pages 29–33.) So listen up: This is equal-opportunity skin-care information.

A good skin-care routine includes cleansing twice a day, usually in the morning before school and at night before bed. Don't get carried away and act like you're scrubbing the tub. Use a soft washcloth, clean gently, and pat dry with a towel.

You don't have to break the bank and buy super-expensive skin products that claim to give you "perfect" skin. Facial soaps and cleansers are made with different ingredients that meet different needs, at different prices. No matter what you use, the product will be on your skin only for a few seconds and then will be rinsed away.

Here are a few of the products you can choose from. Try out a few to see what works best for you:

★ REGULAR BAR SOAPS: You might want to start with one of these, since they cost less than other products. Soaps are made out of animal or vegetable fat; they clean the dirt, oil, sweat, bacteria, and dead cells off your skin. Some experts say that soaps can be harsh and dry out your skin; others say they work fine for most people. Deodorant soaps are a different story, though. They're fine for stifling body odor, but they're too harsh for the skin on your face.

★ SUPERFATTED SOAPS: Just like the name says, these soaps contain fats such as olive oil or cocoa butter to keep skin moist. They're gentler than regular bar soaps, but they leave oils and fats on your skin, even after rinsing. If your skin is oily, you don't need a superfatted soap.

★ TRANSPARENT SOAPS: These are higher in fat than regular bar soaps and may include ingredients like alcohol, sugar, and glycerin. They're mild but may be drying.

★ SOAPLESS (OR DETERGENT) SOAPS: Made from a mixture of petroleum products, these soaps are designed to be mild and work well for most skin types. They rinse off better than other soaps.

★ LIQUID CLEANSERS: These products are made to gently clean skin that's sensitive, dry, or prone to breakouts. Cleansers come in many forms, such as gels, foams, lotions, or creams. You also can find cleansing wipes, which are great to throw in your backpack for touch ups.

You'd think we all live in a desert the way cosmetic companies tell us to rush out and buy their moisturizers because our skin is so desperate for a drink. At your age, you probably have plenty of moisture in your skin, especially in the skin on your face. Because your skin already is moist, using a moisturizer could clog your pores or create oilier skin.

If you have dry or sensitive skin, a moisturizer can help lock in your skin's natural moisture. Moisturizers are also helpful during cold, dry winters and can soothe weather-chapped skin. Just be careful about "glopping" too much moisturizer on your face because it could lead to zits.

You might want to choose a moisturizing lotion instead of a cream, because lotions contain more water and feel lighter. Creams, on the other hand, are designed for very dry skin. If you have acne, don't aggravate it with heavy moisturizers.

## Fact!

Your skin is 70 percent water.

★

Thousands of years ago, Egyptian women moisturized their skin by placing a hunk of scented grease on their heads and letting it melt onto their skin throughout the day.

★

Lanolin, an ingredient in moisturizers, originally starts out as a stinky, waxy product that comes from sheep's fleece.

"I don't like my skin much because sometimes it is really shiny, but sometimes it is dry like paper."
—Sam, 13

These days, you might be more concerned about oil than moisture. Have you heard of the "T-zone"? This term, probably coined by beauty experts, refers to skin that's a combination of dry and oily. It's common to have more oily areas on the forehead, nose, and chin (these zones form a "T" shape). The cheeks are often drier areas. If you have a T-zone, or "combination skin," you don't have to buy one soap for the oily parts and another for the dry ones. You can use one product for your whole face—just find one that works well for you.

TV commercials and magazine ads might tell you that you've got to buy the latest astringent or toner to cut through the oil on your face and firm up your skin. The alcohol and other ingredients in these products can help your skin feel tighter or firmer, but you don't actually get firmer skin out of the deal—just dryer skin and a few less dollars in your pocket. Some of these products contain menthol (an ingredient that can help clear your nose when you have a cold) to give you a tingly feeling on your skin. The truth is, your skin will survive nicely if you forget the astringent and simply clean it well.

Advertisers also want you to buy exfoliating soaps and scrubs that supposedly make your skin softer and smoother. Your skin is tender, right? So you probably wouldn't want to take a wiry dish scrubber to it. That's what these harsh products are like. Some actually use bits of volcanic rock to rub off the outer layer of your skin and allow new cells to come to the surface. (Those dead skin cells would have flaked off naturally in a day or so anyway.) Exfoliating soaps and scrubs can lead to dry, sore skin. A washcloth is a cheaper, softer choice for your face.

You might have seen commercials about people getting "la-dee-dah" facial masks at a spa for the ultimate in pampering. Save your money—and your skin. Facial mask ingredients are designed to harden on your face, and then must be peeled off. The object is to pull off any dirt and dead cells. A mask may dry out your skin, or even kick your oil glands into overdrive to make up for the oil that's stripped away with the mask. Although it won't damage your skin to try a mask once in a while, don't expect miracles. After you remove the product, your face will still be the same face you see in the mirror every day.

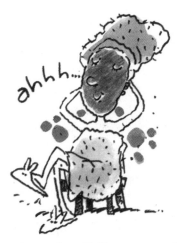

The bottom line? Cleansing your skin with a washcloth and the soap or cleanser of your choice is probably all you need. Just do it twice a day. Follow up with a moisturizer or astringent only if necessary. When in doubt, talk to an adult you trust about a skin-care routine that will work for you.

## SKIN PROBLEMS

No matter who you are, you might have problems with your skin, especially during puberty. No one on earth has ever had (or ever will have) perfect skin. It simply doesn't exist. Television and magazines may lead you to believe otherwise. When you look at actors, models, and other celebrities, it's easy to assume their skin is flawless and they've never had a skin problem in their lives. Not so. They have the benefit of professional makeup and lighting artists to make them look picture-perfect. Take all that away, and these people look more like the rest of us.

### Acne Facts

Who among us hasn't had a pimple? If you can answer, "Yoo-hoo! I've always had perfect skin!" you might belong in the record books, or maybe the zit fairy just hasn't visited you yet. More than 85 percent of teenagers get acne. So, you'll probably have blemishes of some sort before, during, and after puberty—just like everyone else.

The cause of acne is a mystery, but doctors have a pretty good idea about what happens. They think that heredity, stress, and hormones

"My skin breaks out in unbelievable amounts of zits. I keep my skin clean and washed. Is this genetic?"
—Erin, 13

may trigger acne. In other words, your parents and grandparents have something to do with whether your skin is clear or more acne-prone. Hormones play a big role, too.

Remember those oil glands in your skin? When you're a little kid, the glands produce just enough oil to keep your hair and skin soft. As you mature and your hormones start bouncing around, your oil glands kick into high gear and start churning out more oil. If the oil glands become inflamed and the pores get clogged with oil, dead skin cells, and sweat, then bacteria start to grow. When your body tries to get rid of the bacteria, you get *whiteheads, blackheads,* or *pimples* (zits). Here's an explanation of differences between them:

★ WHITEHEADS are pores that have become closed and plugged with oil.

★ BLACKHEADS are plugged pores that haven't closed; pigment has turned the oil black.

★ PIMPLES (or zits) are red, inflamed, plugged pores that sometimes are topped with pus, which forms when the body's white blood cells arrive to kill off bacteria. (When the cells die, they make pus—not a pretty picture.)

Acne can be made worse by stress, illness, medications, and oily lotions. In more severe forms of acne, *cysts* may occur. These large bumps develop deep beneath the skin and may lead to scarring. Cystic acne is hard to treat with over-the-counter medicines, so see a doctor if you have this problem.

If you're of African-American heritage, you'll need to take special care of any acne problems. Because your skin produces pigment faster, it may darken more in areas that become inflamed or injured from breakouts. Treat your skin gently. Use water-based (not oil-based) skin products, which are less likely to cause clogged pores and acne.

# DON'T BELIEVE THE ACNE MYTHS

★ ACNE IS **NOT** CAUSED BY FOODS, SUCH AS CHOCOLATE AND FRENCH FRIES. These foods aren't great for your health, but they don't cause or worsen acne. Some people eat junk foods like these when they're stressed out; coincidentally, stress sometimes triggers blemishes.

★ IF YOUR HAIR TOUCHES YOUR FACE, IT WILL **NOT** CAUSE ACNE. The oil on your hair isn't the problem—it's the oil trapped in clogged pores. However, keeping your hair clean is a good idea.

★ ACNE **DOESN'T** MEAN YOU'RE DIRTY. This myth may have come from the "dirty" appearance of blackheads. The reality is that acne happens to plenty of clean people.

★ IT'S **NOT** TRUE THAT THE MORE YOU WASH YOUR FACE, THE MORE YOU'LL GET RID OF ACNE. You only need to wash your face twice a day to keep it clean. Don't over-scrub your skin with harsh soaps or exfoliating cleansers. You might dry out your skin to the point where you need to apply moisturizers that may clog your pores. It can be a vicious cycle.

This may be only a small comfort, but about 95 percent of people will have acne at some point in their lives, even as adults. It's hard to be objective about how bad your own case of acne is. When it's happening to you, it seems huge.

Although there's no cure for acne, you can find lots of acne-fighting products at any drugstore. Most of these products use ingredients like *sulfur/resorcinol* (kills bacteria), *salicylic acid* (opens clogged pores and clears blackheads), and *benzoyl peroxide* (unclogs pores and kills bacteria). These ingredients may dry out or irritate your skin. If your skin is irritated, stop using the product and try another one.

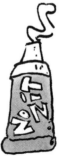

A good skin-care routine can help fight breakouts, too. Here are ten general acne-fighting "rules" to follow:

1. Be gentle to your skin. Wash with *mild* soaps or cleansers.

2. Use oil-free skin products.

3. Avoid astringents, which can be very drying.

4. Don't squeeze or pop pimples. This may cause swelling, skin damage, a bacterial infection, or scarring.

5. Drink lots of water. Much of your skin consists of water, so it functions better when it's hydrated.

6. Avoid being in the kitchen when greasy foods are cooked, if possible. Even though eating greasy foods doesn't cause acne, standing over a pot of hot grease will only put an extra layer of oil on your skin.

7. Protect your skin from sunburn. People used to think that sunlight helped cure acne. But exposure to sunlight can thicken the outer layer of the skin, which may then close the pores and cause further problems.

8. Exercise to help keep your stress levels down (stress triggers acne in some people).

9. Eat a healthy diet. In particular, choose foods and beverages that contain vitamins A, B, C, and E—all of which are good for your skin.

10. Consult a doctor if you have anything other than a mild case of acne.

If you have severe acne, your doctor might prescribe one of several prescription drugs. Choices include antibiotics that you apply to your skin or that are taken in the form of a pill. Or a doctor may recommend drugs called

Retin-A or Accutane. These drugs may have serious side effects, which is why a doctor must prescribe them and check your progress. No drug is an overnight wonder; sometimes, it takes weeks or months to see an improvement.

## The Great Pimple Cover-up

Some people take hiding their pimples really seriously. It's like they think their pimples have to be as top secret as an assignment for the C.I.A. But *everyone* gets zits. It's nothing to be ashamed about.

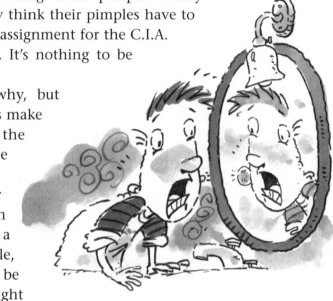

No one knows why, but these pesky blemishes make an appearance at the worst times. Big dance coming up? Need to give a speech to your whole class? Your skin seems to think that's a great time for a pimple, and most likely, it will be one that sticks straight up off your nose.

Picking at the pimple isn't the answer. That's been tried about a million times by millions of other people, and it still doesn't work. Usually, picking at pimples makes them more swollen and red. What can you do instead? Try a tinted acne medication or a concealer stick to tone down the redness. Boys and girls alike can use these products, which you can find in the makeup aisle or the acne medication section at a drugstore. Choose one shade lighter than your skin color, and then dab the concealer on the pimple and lightly blend it into your skin.

Believe it or not, people won't spend all their time looking at a zit or two on your face. The fact is, they're probably too busy thinking about the zits on their *own* faces.

## (Not So) Fun in the Sun

Sun is your skin's worst enemy. Sound extreme? Just check out someone who has spent a lifetime tanning or working outside during the hottest hours of the day. That wrinkly, age-spotted, and leathery look came from the sun.

When the sun's ultraviolet (UV) rays hit your skin, it reacts by producing more melanin as a defense. The darkening is known as a tan. Although our culture makes us believe that a tan is a sign of good health, it's not. It's a sign of skin damage, like a sunburn. Getting a sunburn isn't much different than burning your hand on a skillet or in scalding hot water. A burn is a burn.

If you have skin that's very sensitive to the sun, you know how much a sunburn can hurt. The lighter your coloring, the more careful you need to be in the sun. Even if you tend to tan more than you burn, you're still damaging your skin. People who have darker skin are affected by the sun's UV rays, just as lighter-skinned people are. While it's true that the more melanin you have, the more protected you are from sun damage, you're still at risk. No matter what your skin type or color, WEAR SUNSCREEN!

Sunscreens have been around since 1928, and they come in a variety of strengths and formulas. Sunscreens are rated by the Food and Drug Administration (FDA), and are sorted by their Sun Protection Factor (SPF). An SPF rating of 20 tells you that it would take 20 times as long for you to burn with sunscreen on your skin as it would without it. You should apply sunscreen at least 30 minutes before you go out into the sun, so the product has time to absorb into your skin. Reapply after sweating or getting wet.

It's a great habit to put some sunscreen on your face every day, no matter what the season and even when it's cloudy. Keep some handy in your backpack, so you have it with you whenever you need it.

## Fact!

The sun today is more intense than it was 20 or 30 years ago. Pollution has thinned the sky's ozone layer, which used to soak up more of the sun's ultraviolet rays than it does today.

## Myth!

"You can get a 'base tan' by going to a tanning bed." There's no such thing as a base tan! "Fake baking" even for a few minutes in a tanning bed can be like hours spent in the sun as far as the damage done.

When you repeatedly expose yourself to sun, the rays make your skin fibers loosen, and you get wrinkles later in life. The rays also damage your pigment producers, causing blotchy, toughened skin, freckles, moles, and even skin cancer. Don't want your skin to match that snappy leather jacket? Grab the sunscreen!

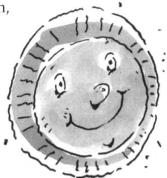

Here's one last thing you can do to keep your skin looking great: Avoid the smoking habit. Ever look at a lifetime smoker's skin? You'll see tiny lines everywhere, especially around the mouth, plus plenty of big wrinkles. If you stay away from cigarettes, you'll save not only your lungs but your skin, too. When you get older, you'll be glad you did.

## THAT FACE LOOKING BACK AT YOU

Pretend you're looking in a mirror. What do you think of yourself? Are you happy with the face looking back at you? Or do you tell yourself you look dorky, ugly, stupid, or some other negative thing?

Maybe looking in the mirror you focus all your attention on one feature:

✱ a nose that seems too big, small, or crooked

✱ those ears that stick out or hug your head too close

✱ oily skin, dry skin, or zits

✱ eyebrows that seem to grow like weeds

✱ skin that's too light, dark, or in-between

Although we all look different, we all have something in common: We get what we get. We're all given different facial features—and we can thank our parents for that. Some of us could go on and on about what's "wrong" with the face staring back at us. The trick is to accept what we've got and make the best of it.

You've probably seen celebrities who've gone a little crazy with plastic surgery and have had their facial features changed (possibly more than once). Some of these people look freaky. Maybe you're dreaming of the day when you can get plastic surgery, too. Think again. For one thing, it's expensive. For another thing, it's painful. Most important, you're fine the way you are.

Right now, your body is going through changes, and so is your face. During puberty, it's normal for your nose and ears to get bigger, or for your face to seem out of proportion. You may feel as if changes are happening almost overnight, or you may see your friends changing and think you still look like a "little kid." Either way, you may feel uncomfortable.

What can you do? The key is not to focus too much on your appearance. Don't spend all your time in front of a mirror or obsess about every change you see. You're more than your looks. You're more than a face. You're an entire person!

## The Makeup Question

If you're a girl, you may be thinking about using makeup. Maybe your friends are starting to wear it, and you'd like to see how makeup might enhance your looks. Most likely, your mom or dad will have an opinion about whether you're at the right age to wear makeup. It's best to talk to a parent before spending several weeks worth of allowance on new cosmetics.

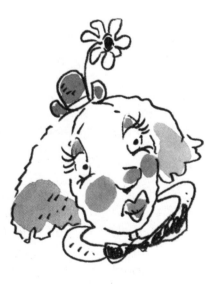

If you decide to try wearing makeup, keep in mind that less is more. You've probably seen girls and women who wear so much makeup they look like they belong in a traveling circus. Too much makeup looks worse than none at all. At your age, you may want to start with just a little blush and lip color in subtle shades of color. If you want to try eye makeup, go for a natural shade of eye shadow, instead of something that shouts for attention. If you want to wear mascara, dab it on lightly so your lashes don't look like a spider's legs.

If you feel you're ready to try a foundation (skin makeup), choose one that closely matches your skin color. Look for a foundation that's sheer, meaning it covers your skin lightly (as opposed to heavy goop that looks like someone put it on with a garden trowel). You may want to dust your skin with a bit of face powder to absorb oil, if needed.

It's important to choose foundations that match your skin type (dry, oily, etc.). Here are some of the different types available:

★ WATER-BASED: These are made with more water than oil, and are best used for dry or normal skin (not oily skin).

★ OIL-BASED: These are made for drier skin to help keep it moist.

★ OIL-FREE: These work best for oily skin, or skin that easily gets clogged pores.

★ POWDER-BASED: Because the powder helps soak up excess oil, these products are best for oily skin.

You'll probably have to experiment with different types of makeup to see what works best for you. Remember to wash the makeup off your face every night before bed, so it won't clog your pores or get in your eyes while you sleep. Use a special eye-makeup remover, instead of washing your eye area with a soap that may be drying. The eye area is the most delicate area of the face, so treat it extra gently.

# MAKEUP THROUGH THE AGES

★ Ancient Egyptian women used dark gray eye paint around their eyes. They thought it made them look beautiful and protected them from harm. The paint also had ingredients that kept flies away.

★ In the 1500s in England, pale skin was highly valued because it showed you were wealthy and didn't have to work outdoors in the sun. Women used a mixture of white lead and vinegar to make their skin look as white as possible; they even painted on fake veins! The lead turned out to be poisonous and made them sick.

★ In Japan, Kabuki dancers painted their faces totally white and then drew on eyebrows and lips with red and black makeup.

★ For thousands of years, people have used the red dye of the henna plant to decorate their arms, hands, legs, and feet with ornamental patterns. Originating in the Middle East and North Africa, the custom was used to make women beautiful and bring good luck. At weddings, even the grooms were decorated.

## Your Ears and Eyes

One of the most noticeable features on your face is your eyes. When was the last time you had them checked? At your age, your eyes, like all your other parts, might start to change. If you squint while looking at the blackboard or have headaches after you read, get checked by an optometrist (eye specialist). You may need to wear glasses. If you already have glasses but you're still squinting, your prescription may be outdated.

These days, there are lots of cool glasses to choose from, in all styles and colors. Are you worried about how you'll look in a pair of frames? Most people feel anxious at first. Sure, glasses will change your looks, but more importantly they'll change how you see the world: clearly and in focus!

If you get glasses, remember to keep them clean. (Think of all the dirt and skin oil your glasses collect each day.) Rinse them daily in warm water and mild dish soap, or use a special eyeglass cleaner. Rub the lenses and frames gently with a soft cloth that won't scratch (100 percent cotton cloth is best). Store your glasses in their case to keep them clean and to prevent them from getting broken.

Maybe you're ready for contact lenses. They can be a great option, especially if you play sports and don't want to wear glasses on the field or court. See an eye doctor to talk about whether these lenses are right for you. Contact lenses are a big responsibility, because you have to clean them and take care of them every day. Some people get grossed out about the idea of touching their eyes while putting the lenses in, so think about whether you can handle that task.

Like your eyes, your ears need special care. Ever hear the saying, "Don't stick anything in your ear smaller than your elbow?" As weird as it sounds, it's true. You'd be surprised at the strange things people stick in their ears to clean them: car keys, pen lids, hairpins, pencil tips. Even cotton swabs shouldn't go in your ears—of course, the companies that sell the swabs want you to think it's necessary. Cotton swabs can harm your eardrums when you poke them around in your ears. In fact, the swabs may actually pack the wax in, rather than clean it out.

If you can't use a cotton swab, how should you clean your ears? Use a damp washcloth. A simple wipe on the outside of your ears is enough.

But let's back up a minute. Why do we have earwax anyway? Does it have a purpose, besides looking kind of gross? Like most other disgusting things our bodies produce (snot, for example), earwax is there for a reason. It's full of helpful chemicals that kill germs. Earwax also traps

## Fact!

Maybe you've wondered about that crusty stuff around your eyes when you wake up in the morning? Even though you quit blinking when you're asleep, the fluids in your eyes keep on oozing. They seep out from your eyelids and dry out overnight.

★

Archeologists have found "earspoons" that were used by Vikings to clean their ears. Made of bone, ivory or metal, some earspoons were so ornamental that women wore them hanging from their jewelry.

★

Earwax acts like a tiny parka, warming the air in your ears.

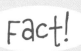

**Fact!**

No one knows why but people of different races have different looking earwax. Most Hispanics, Caucasians, and African Americans have wet, brownish earwax. Asians and Native Americans have dry, gray earwax.

dirt and the occasional bug. So, your ears are self-cleaning. The wax catches its "prey," flakes off, and falls out of your ears on a regular basis.

It *is* possible to get wax buildup. You'll know you have a problem if your ear feels clogged and uncomfortable. There are eardrops available to dissolve the wax so it can be washed out.

## Facial Hair (Some Want It, Some Don't)

Maybe you've noticed new hairs springing up on your face. How you feel about that depends, in part, on whether you're a girl or a boy.

During puberty, boys start to get hair on their upper lip. Many boys are happy about this event, because it means it's nearly time to shave. They see this as a sign of growing up. On the other hand, some boys aren't too happy about getting facial hair at a young age and may feel self-conscious. Whether you get the hair late or early is a result of heredity. Talk to your dad or grandfather about their experiences to get an idea of what you can expect.

Usually, male facial hair begins with the "peach fuzz" mustache stage. The hair is very light and thin, like the fuzzy coating on a peach. Gradually, the hair begins to fill

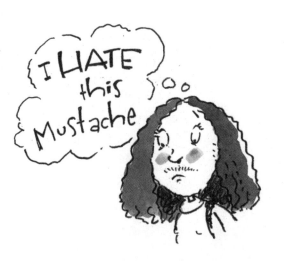

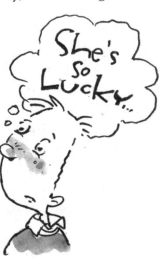

out the mustache area, and then grows on the cheeks, on the sideburn area, and under the lower lip. The lighter hair usually becomes darker and thicker. None of this happens overnight. Be patient if your facial hair is being "shy" about making its appearance. In time, you'll catch up to other boys whose hair may grow faster.

At some point, you'll be ready for your first shave. When that day comes, you'll need to decide whether you want to use an electric shaver or a blade razor. The electric ones are more expensive and won't shave you as close as the blade kind. But they also won't cut you as easily, and you won't have to keep changing blades.

# TIPS FOR SHAVING WITH BLADE RAZORS

★ Wet the skin with warm water to open the pores.

★ Use a thin coat of shaving foam or gel. Pick one that's mild on the skin.

★ Use a sharp razor. Go easy when you shave, instead of scraping or pressing too hard.

★ Rinse the blade as you go, clearing it for a better cut.

★ Rinse your face with warm water after you're done.

If you're of African-American heritage and/or you have curly hair, you may be more likely to get ingrown hairs. This means your hairs often grow back down into

## Fact!

While you might think the hair on your head grows fast, it doesn't compare at all to how fast a man's beard grows. If the average guy never trimmed his beard, he'd have to tie it up and throw it over his shoulder to keep from stepping on it.

★

In America, people spend an average of 3,500 hours of their lives shaving.

**Myth!**

"Waxed hair won't grow back." Wrong! It *will* grow back, but it may be softer and more sparse.

your skin, creating a bump. Shaving in the direction of the hair growth can help prevent this. So can using a washcloth to loosen hairs before they curl inward.

After you finish shaving, pat your face dry (don't rub hard). You can use an after-shave lotion if you want. Avoid alcohol-based shaving lotions, since they can feel like liquid fire after you've shaved (think alcohol poured on a popped blister). Some lotions are made for sensitive skin; they treat it gently and help put some moisture back in.

When *girls* see hairs sprouting above their upper lip, it's a whole different story. They usually aren't too happy about it. It's common for girls who have darker or heavier body hair to see hair on their upper lip or even on their chin. Some use facial-hair bleach to lighten the hairs. Others pluck them with tweezers. Others remove hairs using waxes. And some just don't do anything about it at all.

Waxing isn't for the faint of heart. It involves applying warm, melted wax to your skin, placing a cloth or paper strip over it, and quickly pulling it off. (Your hairs come off with the strip.) The advantage: the hairs may be gone for weeks. The disadvantage: redness, irritation, and pain. If you're going to try this, you might want to wait till the weekend, so you don't have to go to school the next day with red, irritated skin.

If these methods don't work for you and your facial hair really bothers you, you could look into electrolysis or laser hair removal, both of which must be done by a professional. Electrolysis uses electric pulses to zap each hair. Laser treatments use pulses of light to stop hair production for a few weeks. These last two methods are expensive, and may not be a permanent fix. Talk with a parent about your feelings about facial hair before you try any of these hair-removal methods.

Whether you're a girl or a boy, you might notice your eyebrows getting darker, thicker, and bushier—another sign of puberty. Sometimes, the growth is so heavy that you almost look as if you've got one eyebrow growing across the top of your face (also known as a "uni-brow"). You can tweeze your eyebrows to help tame them. The first time you tweeze the hairs, your eyes may water. You'll get used to the feeling once you've tweezed a few times.

As you can see, we humans go through a lot to keep ourselves healthy and looking good. We shave and pluck; we wash and moisturize; we invest in all sorts of anti-pimple products. And we stare into mirrors checking ourselves out. We often wonder whether we look "good enough." If you're in doubt about your appearance, it may help to remember that lots of people your age are in the same situation.

⭐ ⭐ ⭐

There are certain parts of your appearance that you can't control: the color of your skin, the shape of your ears, or the size of your nose. It's best to accept these parts of yourself and get on with your life. However, you *can* control how you care for your skin. You also can choose a great pair of glasses or wear a little makeup if it makes you feel better. These small efforts can improve your appearance.

Did you know that there's one sure-fire way to put your best face forward? Smile! A smile can do wonders for your appearance and make you feel good inside. There's no doubt that people respond more positively to a smile than a frown or a scowl. In the next chapter, you'll learn about keeping your smile as bright as it possibly can be.

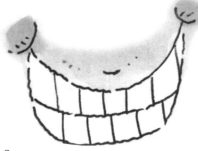

**Fact!**

Why *do* we have eyebrows? They act like little gutters, diverting water or sweat from our eyes. Eyebrows also are very useful when "reading" other people's moods.

⭐

Next time you look at the famous painting of the Mona Lisa, check out her smooth brow. In the Renaissance period in Italy, many women shaved off their eyebrows.

# CHAPTER 3

# Your MOUTH (An Amusement Park for Germs)

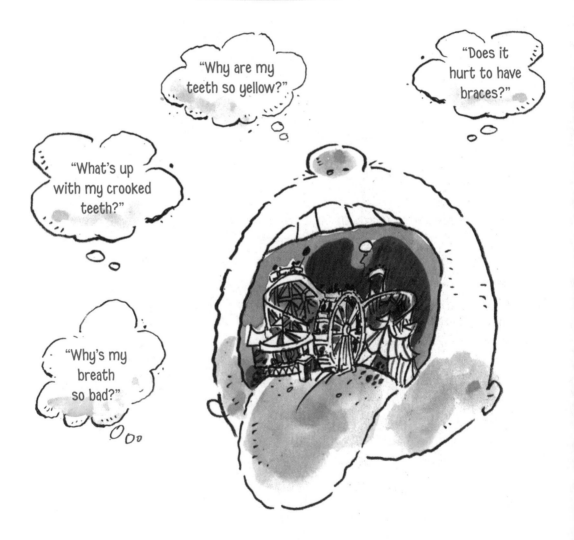

"Why are my teeth so yellow?"

"Does it hurt to have braces?"

"What's up with my crooked teeth?"

"Why's my breath so bad?"

44

$\mathcal{S}$uppose you're watching a music awards show on TV. Your favorite recording artist is onstage, belting out her latest hit song, and the camera zooms in on her blindingly white teeth—perfectly straight, not a filling in sight. Maybe you start to wonder why your own "pearly whites" aren't quite so pearly white as hers. Why does everyone on television seem to have a perfect smile, while the rest of us have, well, something else?

I'll let you in on a few secrets. First, most celebrities go to great lengths to get their gorgeous smiles. Pricey cosmetic dentistry can produce straight, white teeth that look beautifully fresh and clean. But guess what? Celebrities are human like the rest of us, which means their mouths—like yours—are swarming with millions of germs. Bacteria love the warm, moist environment of the human mouth. (For more on bacteria, see page 25.) Here, bacteria have a great time exploring your teeth and gums. If you let that bacteria run wild, big problems can result. That's why it's so important to take care of your mouth. Read on to learn how.

## YOUR TERRIFIC TEETH

Most of us take our teeth for granted. They're there when we need to crunch a potato chip, mow the kernels off an ear of corn, or chomp our favorite gum. Just imagine what life would be like *without* your teeth. Suppose you had to wear false teeth like some elderly people do, and take out your teeth every night before bed. Your face would get that caved-in look without your teeth there to maintain the shape of your face. Plus, it would be harder for you to talk, because your teeth help you speak clearly.

When you were a little kid, the thought of losing your baby teeth was probably exciting. You couldn't wait to yank out each tooth and put it under your pillow for the Tooth Fairy. You may have been excited to see your "big" teeth (permanent teeth) come in. And BIG they were. Permanent teeth tend to look huge on most kids because their faces still have a lot of growing to do.

In addition to your 28 permanent teeth, you may get four wisdom teeth later in life. These teeth tend to show up when you're anywhere from eighteen to forty—old enough, supposedly, to be wise. Your permanent teeth are just that—permanent. That's all you get for the rest of your

By the time you're about 11, you'll complete the process of losing all 20 of your baby teeth and getting your 28 permanent teeth.

★

You may think you've got lots of teeth. But compared to some animals, humans are "lightweights." Alligators can have as many as 2,000 teeth throughout their lifetime; they continually lose and grow new teeth, just as sharks do.

life. If you live to be eighty or so, your teeth will need to last that long. If you don't want to lose them in your old age, take care of them now while you're young and keep up the healthy habits all your life.

Different teeth are designed to do different jobs. Your *incisors,* or front teeth, are sharp so they can slice the food you eat. Your *canines* are the pointy teeth that look somewhat like a dog's fangs; these teeth help tear food up. Way in the back of your mouth, you've got *molars,* which are wider and can grind food. Because molars have lots of grooves and pits, they're more likely to get tooth decay than other teeth.

Your teeth are tough so that you're able to chew meat and vegetables. In fact, the *enamel,* or the outside covering of your teeth, is the hardest substance in your body—even harder than bone. *Dentin,* a hard yellow substance, makes up the inside of your teeth. Deep down inside lies the *pulp*—the soft part that's full of blood vessels and nerves. These nerves send messages to your brain to tell you how hard to bite into foods. The nerves also let you know in a hurry if you've got a broken or rotten tooth.

## The Truth About Tooth Decay

It's a good thing we don't carry around microscopes, because we probably wouldn't want to see the microorganisms that share our personal space. These tiny creatures just love our mouths, where the temperature's constant, the humidity level is high, and the "amusement park" is always open.

Not surprisingly, there are interesting places in your mouth for these creatures to hang out—between your teeth, along your gum line, in the crevices of your tongue, and on the roof of your mouth. Some of these microorganisms help break down foods and fight off bad bacteria. It's those other ones you need to watch out for—the ones that eat away at your tooth enamel.

You've probably heard your dentist or another adult talk about *plaque.* This sticky coating develops on your teeth and can build up over time. If you don't brush it away after meals, it hardens into a substance called *tartar* (not the tartar sauce you put on fish sticks). While your teeth seem smooth, there actually are lots of crevices where the plaque and tartar build up. Plaque is soft and sticky; tartar is the hard stuff your dentist has to scrape off with special dental tools.

You can see and feel the plaque on your teeth right now, if you want to. Take your fingernail or a toothpick and carefully scrape a tooth around your gum line. That white, gooey stuff that comes off is plaque. To feel the coating of plaque on your teeth, run your tongue over your teeth and check out the rough sensation. Then take a small piece of cloth and rub it over your teeth for about ten seconds. Feel your teeth with your tongue again. This time, they should be much smoother. That's because you've removed some plaque with the cloth.

When you have a buildup of plaque and tartar, you're at risk for a *cavity,* or a hole in your tooth. Here's how it happens: The sugars in the foods you eat mix with bacteria in your mouth, and acid is created. Your *saliva,* or spit, is supposed to neutralize the acid, but it can't do the job if the acid is locked inside a layer of plaque. The more sugar you consume, the more acid there is around your teeth.

The acid starts to eat away at your tooth enamel, and soon you're on your way to a cavity. A tiny hole is created, one that eventually reaches the dentin. The acid starts to attack the nerves, and you start to feel some pain. After a while, the acid may work its way into the soft pulp of your tooth, and you get a real zinger of a toothache. If cavities are caught early (before they reach the pulp), they can be fixed with a small filling. Getting a filling means a dentist has to drill out the decayed part of the tooth, and

**Fact!**

Some of the good "creatures" in your mouth are called tooth amoebas, which look like blobs of jelly. They help your teeth by feeding on bacteria and leftover food.

then fill it in with a hard substance (usually a mixture of silver and other metals). Fillings can be tiny or fill almost a whole tooth.

These days, dentists are seeing more patients who have lots of teeth to fill. The reason? Soda pop. Not only do people drink colas and other soft drinks more often than ever before, but they drink *lots* of them. In fact, some convenience stores sell cups that can hold as much as 60 ounces of soda at once. That's equal to the amount in five cans!

Before you reach for a soft drink, consider these facts:

✹ The average can of soda contains 10 teaspoons of sugar.

✹ The average American drinks 56 gallons of soda in a year.

✹ Sodas also contain tooth-damaging acids. If you were to soak a penny overnight in cola, the next morning you'd find that the acids in the cola had cleaned the money. Think what those acids can do to your tooth enamel.

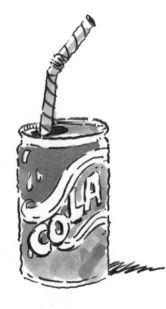

✹ After you drink sugar, acids attack your teeth for about 30 minutes.

Your school may have soda machines available, making it easier to buy these products. But once you get into the habit of drinking lots of pop, the habit can be hard to break. Soon your body will start to crave the sugar and caffeine. A better choice when you're thirsty? Milk, fruit juice, or water.

# HOW TO HAVE A HEALTHY SMILE

Whether or not you'll need lots of fillings may depend on the type of teeth your parents have. Studies have shown that, while taking good care of your teeth is always important, you might inherit teeth that either are naturally strong or tend to need dental work. Still, you have the power to help your teeth be as strong and healthy as possible. Eating less sugar is a good start, and learning to brush and floss your teeth correctly is key.

Brushing your teeth not only removes food particles but also gets rid of plaque. So brush, brush, brush! Dentists recommend that you give your teeth a good brushing at least twice a day. Brush for *two minutes* to make sure you do a thorough job. You may want to keep a special timer in the bathroom, so you brush for the recommended amount of time.

Here are a few tips to get the most out of brushing:

✱ Use a small toothbrush with medium bristles. Replace your toothbrush every three or four months, or when it starts to look worn.

✱ Use a circular motion when you brush. Try to clean in between your teeth, too.

✱ Don't scrub too hard, or you might wear grooves in your tooth enamel.

✱ Some dentists recommend using powered toothbrushes and water irrigators, which shoot jets of water along your gum line to blow out food particles. However, the American Dental Association (ADA) says that regular toothbrushes are just as good as the electric ones, if you do a good job when brushing. (That doesn't mean you get to be lazy about brushing with a powered toothbrush. You still have to work at it!)

Fact!

Some of the first human toothbrushes were twigs. People chewed twigs to scrape the plaque off their teeth; oils from the wood killed bacteria.

✱

Throughout history, dentures (fake teeth) have been made of bone, gold, ivory, porcelain, or the teeth of animals and humans. Human teeth often were gathered from dead soldiers on battlefields.

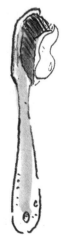

★ When buying a toothbrush (or any dental product), look for the ADA Seal of Acceptance on it.

★ Choose toothpaste that contains fluoride (most brands do). Fluoride strengthens tooth enamel and fights plaque. Use only a pea-sized blob of toothpaste, and avoid swallowing it when you brush.

★ Be sure to brush your tongue, too.

Follow up with flossing. Dental floss is specially designed to get at that hard-to-reach plaque between your teeth. Dentists recommend that you floss at least once a day. Unwaxed floss grabs more plaque from between your teeth than the waxed kind, but some people prefer the smoother texture of waxed dental floss. See what works for you.

Taking good care of your teeth now may prevent gum disease later in life. Gum disease happens when bacteria from plaque and tartar infects your gums. Your gums begin to pull away from your teeth, giving bacteria more room to grow. Gum disease can be prevented if you do a good job of brushing and flossing your teeth and visit a dentist regularly.

Going to the dentist probably doesn't rate as one of your favorite activities. But at least you don't live during the Middle Ages, a time when *barbers* were the ones practicing dentistry! (You could get a haircut and your teeth pulled at the same time.) A few hundred years ago, dental technology had improved but not by much. Dentists didn't know how to fix decayed teeth, so they simply pulled them. Sometimes they'd have musicians play loud music, so people in the street couldn't hear the patient's screams of pain. Back then, they didn't have the pain-killers we have today.

The fact is dentists actually can save you from a lot of pain. Your dentist can take X-rays to look inside your teeth and gums, and catch cavities early. At the dentist's office, you also can have your teeth cleaned by a professional. Get a dental checkup every six months, if possible. Remember, the dentist is there to help you care for the teeth you plan to have for your whole life.

Dental care isn't always affordable for some families. You can contact your state's Dental Society to find out about low-cost programs that may be available in your area. Another option is finding a dental college, which may charge less than a private dentist's office. Your Dental Society can help you locate dental colleges in your area.

One final way to keep your teeth in good shape is to wear a mouth guard when you play sports. There are three types of mouth guards: *custom-made, mouth-formed,* and *ready-made.* The custom-made mouth guard is designed by your dentist after he or she makes an impression of your teeth; it gives you the best protection. The mouth-formed type (also called a "boil and bite") is available at most sporting goods stores; you bite into a mouth guard that's been softened in boiling water and then let it harden over your teeth. Ready-made mouth guards are the cheapest kind, but they don't protect you as well as other ones because they don't conform to the unique shape of your teeth. No matter what kind of mouth guard you choose, it will take some getting used to. It sure beats having a tooth knocked out, though!

## Eat Right for a Healthy Bite

Archeologists have uncovered skulls of people who lived thousands of years ago, and many of those ancient people had all their teeth all their lives. That's probably because they weren't sitting around eating candy bars or sucking on hard candies. They didn't have access to the sugary foods that create tooth decay.

Let's face it: Most of us love to eat sugar. Maybe you have what's known as a "sweet tooth"? It's hard to pass up cookies, brownies, candy, doughnuts, and other sweet treats. But eating fewer of these items will help your teeth now and down the road. You don't have to give up sweets altogether; just limit them. Try to say no to sodas, sugary frozen drinks, and powdered drink mixes as well (all of them contain sugar).

You know the harm sugar can do, but there are other cavity-producers that might surprise you. Foods like cereal and crackers can create tooth decay. So can sticky foods such as raisins and granola bars. The longer they stick to your teeth, the more damage they can do.

High-fiber foods such as fruits and vegetables, on the other hand, can help clean your teeth. These foods send out a call to your salivary glands to start kicking out the spit (the saliva helps neutralize acid that eats away at your teeth). Fruits and veggies leave a coating of moisture on your teeth, which helps keep away stains and bacteria. You also can choose foods that are rich in calcium, such as yogurt and cheese; they're good for your teeth because they strengthen your tooth enamel.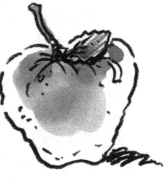

# HOW TO BEAT THE SWEETS

1. Brush and floss after every meal or snack. At the very least, brush twice a day and floss once. You can't exactly whip out your toothbrush every time you put food in your mouth, of course. But you can keep a spare toothbrush and some toothpaste in your locker or backpack for when you do get a chance to brush.

2. Only eat sweets at times when you can brush your teeth afterward.

3. If you can't brush right after eating sweets, rinse your mouth with water afterward instead. Or finish with a piece of cheese or some apple slices to help your saliva wash away the acids that collect on your teeth.

4. Use a straw to drink sweet liquids, so they're less likely to touch your teeth.

## wANt whiter Teeth?

Flip through the pages of any teen magazine, and you'll see a lot of gleaming white teeth. When you look at your own in the mirror, they may not seem so bright. In fact, they might look a bit yellow in comparison. That's because you probably haven't had cosmetic dentistry to whiten and brighten your teeth, while most models have.

Some people's tooth enamel naturally looks more yellow than other people's. So don't compare your teeth to your best friend's or anyone else's. The best you can do is to work with what you've got. If you want whiter teeth, then brush and floss regularly. You may want to buy a whitening toothpaste or, every so often, brush with baking soda (look for it in the kitchen cupboard). You also can limit drinks that stain teeth (particularly cola, coffee, or tea).

Avoid tobacco products, too. Studies have shown that about 15 percent of middle-school students have used some type of tobacco in the past year; about 35 percent of high school students have. Fast forward and check out these young smokers as adults: If you were to open their mouths, you'd find stained teeth and raw-looking gums, not to mention stinky breath. Smokeless or chewing tobacco causes these kinds of problems, too. Plus, tobacco companies add sugar to these products to make them taste better, adding more risk of tooth decay.

## Brace Yourself for Braces

Metal Mouth. Jaws. Tinsel Teeth. Brace Face. You've heard the names for people who have braces. If you're scared of having a mouth full of metal, you're not alone. Braces can be a sensitive issue. You may wonder if people will tease you. You may think braces will slow down your

"You could call me a 'metal mouth.' I have a 'lip bumper' that blocks the pressure on my front teeth. I will get 'train tracks' in sixth grade."
—Rachel, 10

social life, especially if you need to wear them for several years. These questions and worries are normal. Just about everyone who gets braces feels nervous at first.

Here's how braces work: Metal bands are cemented on each tooth, and wires are used to connect them. An orthodontist tightens and loosens the wires as needed to move the teeth 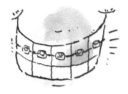 into proper alignment. The sockets that hold the teeth are forced to move along the jawbone, and new bone grows in the space that's left. All this shifting can cause a sore mouth at times, especially when the braces are adjusted.

There are other orthodontic appliances you might need as well. For example, you might have to wear a headgear to make your teeth move into position faster. You may need a "lip bumper" to keep your lips from putting too much pressure on your front teeth. Or you might require a retainer—a piece of plastic and metal that fits into your mouth to help hold your teeth in place, usually after you get your braces removed. Every person has a different experience in what type of orthodontic work is needed and how long the process takes.

Keep in mind that you're responsible for using any of the devices your orthodontist provides. A headgear isn't much fun, but you need to wear it if you have one. Same goes for a retainer. Wouldn't you hate it if, after wearing braces for a year or two, your newly straightened teeth begin to get crooked again *because you didn't wear your retainer?* Don't let that happen!

It's important to take good care of these devices when you have them. Maybe you're familiar with the sight of some kid digging through the cafeteria garbage, desperately trying to find a lost retainer? No fun. Store your retainer in its case when you're not wearing it to prevent that kind of mistake.

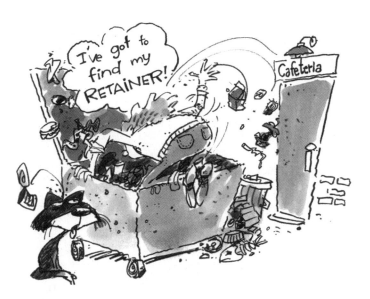

Keeping your retainer clean is essential because it spends so much time in your (germ-filled) mouth. Take the retainer out and brush it with your toothbrush and toothpaste at least twice a day—in the morning and at bedtime—to kill germs. You also can soak it in mouthwash or a denture cleanser, if you want.

You probably know that it's important to keep braces clean, too. But this isn't always easy. (Ever see someone with braces smile after eating? A little tater tot here, a bit of broccoli there.) Brushing after meals helps remove these food particles and clean out all the nooks and crannies that are the perfect places for bacteria to hide. In fact, brushing at least four times a day (in the morning, after lunch or school, after supper, and at bedtime) is the best way to keep braces clean. Ask your orthodontist about special toothbrushes and water irrigators that can help you keep your teeth as clean as possible.

Flossing your teeth when you have braces is tricky. You can buy dental floss "threaders" that help you poke the floss under the wires and between your teeth. Be gentle so you don't damage the wires or hurt your gums.

Orthodontists advise patients to have their teeth professionally cleaned every three months while they have braces. It's also wise to limit hard or sticky foods—popcorn, ice, nuts, gum, taffy, caramels, raisins—that might damage your braces or get caught in your teeth.

About 70 percent of teens wear braces, so if you get braces someday, you definitely won't be alone. Instead of worrying about braces, try to keep your eye on the prize: a set of straight teeth. Focusing on this goal can make the time you wear braces seem like less of a pain.

## KISS BAD BREATH GOOD-BYE

Bad breath ranks high as something that worries kids your age—at least according to the kids I've visited in schools during presentations. Many of them have said they're worried about their breath and don't know what to do.

You're probably more clued into bad breath now than you were when you were little. It's not that you used to be clueless—your breath just wasn't a big deal back then. These days, you're probably more interested in the impression you're making on others. You want fresh breath when you're talking to people.

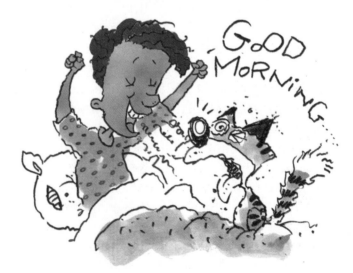

You can take the Breath Test right now. Just put your palm in front of your face, breathe out through your mouth, and then quickly breathe in through your nose. Did you get a whiff? How was it?

If you're reading this first thing in the morning, your breath probably isn't at its best. No one wakes up with a clean, fresh mouth because germs and odors collect in there overnight. At other times of the day, you might have bad breath from eating onions or garlic, or simply because it's been a while since you last brushed your teeth.

If you take good care of your teeth by regularly brushing and flossing, you shouldn't have a constant problem with bad breath. Think about whether you're taking good care of your mouth. If you notice you get bad breath during school, it might be because you're eating meals and snacks but not brushing afterward. Keep a toothbrush and toothpaste in your backpack, or stock up on breath mints and sugarless gum. If you notice you have bad breath fairly often, ask yourself whether you're brushing and flossing well enough. At your age, your mom or dad won't be standing over you to make sure you're brushing adequately. It's up to you to do the job.

You may want to try a mouthwash to tame your bad breath. Mouthwash is supposed to kill bacteria, swish bits of food out of your teeth, and give you that minty-fresh feeling. But not all mouthwashes are created equal. Look for the ADA Seal of Approval on the product you choose, so you know it's recommended by dental experts.

Sometimes, a mouthwash may hide the signs of a dental problem. Bad breath and an icky taste in your mouth might be symptoms of a dental condition that could end up being serious. So don't keep pouring on the "Stink-Be-Gone" if your breath is a constant problem. If you notice people holding their breath when you talk, or if your dog slinks away every time you try to kiss him, you might

"I hate it when I have bad breath. It seems like you can brush your teeth 2,000 times, but your breath still smells very, very, very bad."
—Michael, 11

need to see a dentist. Your dentist can check out your mouth and recommend a way to fight bad breath. If your dentist says that your mouth is healthy, you may need to see a doctor to check out possible medical causes of bad breath.

# Don't Forget Your Lips

Your lips are the doorway to your mouth, so to speak. They help you eat, talk, and kiss. Kissing might be something you're wondering more about lately. If kissing is on your mind, mouth care may seem more important than ever. You may be concerned about kissing with bad breath (yuck), kissing with braces (ouch), or kissing someone who smokes (oh, gross). Maybe you never thought of your lips as important—but they are.

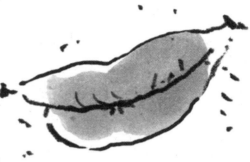

Have you noticed that your lips are cracked, dry, or chapped? Maybe you're a lip licker. In other words, you lick your lips a lot when you're nervous or bored. Maybe you're a lip biter, and you chew your lips when you're concentrating. These habits may not be noticeable until your lips show signs of wear and tear. Spending time in the sun and wind also may lead to chapped lips. You can buy lip balms or petroleum jelly to moisten your lips. It helps to drink more water, too.

Maybe you get small, reddish blisters on your lips every so often. If they tingle and burn, they're probably cold sores. Cold sores are caused by viruses and can be spread by kissing, or even just by sharing a drink with someone. A cold sore will heal on its own, but you can speed up the healing process by using a cold-sore medication that you dab on your lips.

As long as we're on the subject of lips, let's talk about lip piercing. You're too young to do this now, but you may be thinking about it for the future. If so, think about all of the dangers. Your mouth is naturally filled with millions of bacteria, and when you pierce any part of it (your lips, your tongue), you create an open wound for bacteria to hop into. You could end up with a nasty infection, nerve damage, or other problems.

⭐  ⭐  ⭐

With just a little effort, you can take care of your mouth—on the outside and on the inside. If you do, you'll feel better. Who needs chapped lips, bad breath, or tooth decay? Not you. Just spending a few minutes a day brushing and flossing can make a big difference. So can breaking the lip-licking, lip-biting habit. When your mouth is healthy, you'll feel more confident about talking to people. And you'll have a better smile to show the world.

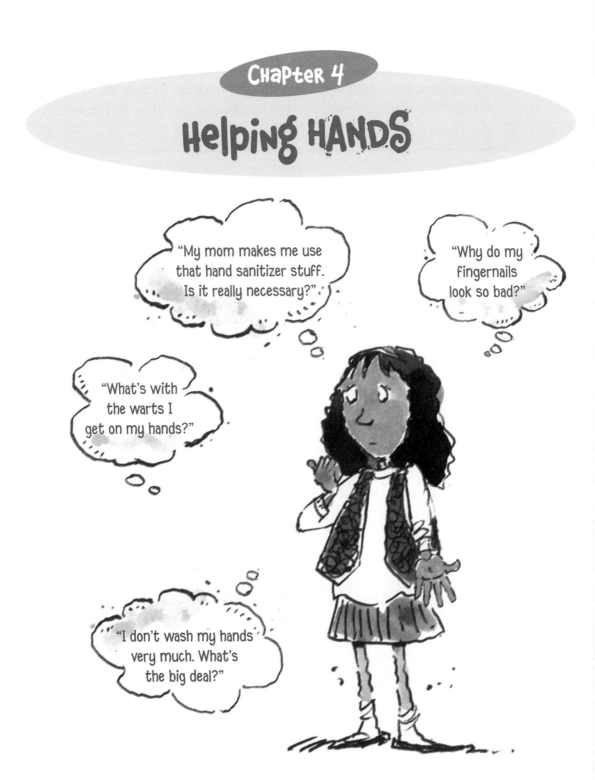

**M**aybe you've heard about people who have a disorder that makes them wash their hands a hundred times a day. They're so afraid of germs, they scrub until their skin is raw. While you don't have to be that freaked out about germs, it doesn't hurt to give them some more thought. Germs are crawling all over your hands right now. If you're biting your nails while you read, you're putting those germs straight into your mouth. Some of those germs can make you sick.

This chapter is all about keeping your hands neat and clean, and why it matters. No one expects you to have the hands of a "hand model"—but walking around with enough dirt under your nails to grow plants in isn't a great idea either. Your hands say something about you. With a little effort, they can say you're someone who's neat and clean.

## WASH GERMS DOWN THE DRAIN

So, why are some people so worked into a lather about washing hands anyway? In your lifetime, your parents probably have told you to wash your hands more times than you can count. You hear about hand washing from doctors, nurses, and teachers, too. What's so important about clean hands?

Think about your hands: they're your tools, and you use them constantly. You rely on your hands when typing at a computer keyboard, catching a ball, eating your lunch, blowing your nose, opening your locker, playing a musical instrument, holding onto a banister, putting on your shoes, cleaning out the cat's litter box, and so on. Now consider all the things you touch when you use your hands.

Suppose you could rub a cotton swab on any object you touch (a computer mouse, a doorknob), and then

## Fact!

Ever wonder why your fingers wrinkle when they get wet? The tough skin on those digits has nowhere to stretch out when it soaks up water, so it folds into wrinkles.

★

The first doctor known for telling people the importance of washing hands and cleaning fingernails was Ignaz Semmelweis, a Hungarian obstetrician, in 1847. Before he stopped them, medical students would go directly from dissecting dead bodies to delivering babies—without washing their hands.

★

There are 206 bones in the human body, 54 of which are in the hands.

A cold-causing rhinovirus (in Greek, *rhin* means nose) can live for up to 3 hours outside the nose on objects or skin.

send the sample out to a lab. What do you think the lab workers would find? Germs, of course. Germs are everywhere. They're floating in the air and hovering on surfaces. Once they get inside you, germs multiply like crazy.

You never know what kinds of germs may be lurking around the corner. When you touch them with your hands, the germs may end up inside you. You introduce germs into your body every day by rubbing your eyes, wiping your nose, or chewing on your fingernails. Luckily, soap and water can cut those germs loose and send them down the drain. Health experts at the Centers for Disease Control say that hand washing is the number one thing you can do to prevent the spread of infection.

You may be thinking, "Our home is pretty clean, I'm not worried about germs." Think again. Just because germs can't be seen doesn't mean they aren't there. Even the cleanest homes are breeding grounds for germs. So are the public places you visit every day: your school, the bus, the library, and the store, for example.

Not to put too fine a point on it, but consider how dirty these public places may be. Suppose a classmate of yours goes into the bathroom and—let's just come right out and say it—he poops. After he wipes, he may have microscopic bits of poop on his hands. Now suppose he forgets to wash his hands, and he opens the bathroom door. What's left on the door handle? You guessed it.

Now suppose you come along and grab that same door handle. You've just contaminated your hand with some nasty germs. You go back to your desk, and while listening to your teacher, you notice you have a hangnail. You decide to trim it with your teeth. Oops, your finger's not the only thing that just went into your mouth! In case you're not grossed out enough: The bacteria from feces can live inside your body without hurting you, but when lots of this bacteria builds up, you can get sick with diarrhea.

The human body has the power to fight off a lot of germs. If it didn't, people would be sick all the time. But why take the chance of getting sick with diarrhea or a cold? By simply washing your hands, you wash away germs that your body doesn't really want or need. It's that easy.

# THE RISKS OF NOT WASHING YOUR HANDS

* You could get a cold, the flu, or an upset stomach from germs.

* You could get a food-related illness after touching raw meat, eggs, or poultry. (You might also get sick if someone who's preparing the food doesn't wash his or her hands.)

* You could get a Salmonella infection from a pet reptile. Most reptiles carry the bacteria called Salmonella, which can be found on their skin, in their cages, and on things they touch. Wash your hands well after touching a reptile, and if you let one swim in your bathtub, scrub it out afterward.

## Hand-washing "How-tos"

You may think it sounds loopy to tell you how to wash your hands at your age, but many people do a pitiful job of it. Some studies have shown that even doctors and nurses could use a refresher on hand washing. In a 1992 study reported in the *New England Journal of Medicine* (a magazine for people in the medical field), researchers found that, in a hospital intensive care unit, only 30 to 48 percent of the staffers were washing their hands.

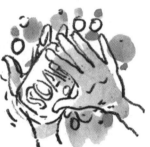

Apparently, lots of people have forgotten their parents' lectures on washing their hands after using the restroom. In a recent study by the

American Society of Microbiology's Clean Hands Campaign, undercover observers went into public restrooms in New York City, Atlanta, New Orleans, Chicago, and San Francisco. After watching close to 8,000 people without being too obvious about what they were doing (a person can only comb their hair for so long), the observers found that plenty of those restroom-users completely forgot about hand washing.

In Atlanta, for example, close to 65 percent of the men who were secretly watched walked right on past the bathroom sinks. Although about 95 percent of people say they wash their hands after using the restroom, 33 percent don't wash up. That's alarming because those "non-washers" leave their germs on surfaces we all touch.

Here's the lowdown on washing your hands thoroughly:

1. Wet your hands with warm water and apply soap. (You don't need a ton of it—a squirt from a soap pump will do the job.)

2. Turn off the water while you scrub, so you don't waste water. Scrub vigorously (as if you were removing a sticky mixture of bacon grease and flour).

3. Wash your palms, the tops of your hands, in between your fingers, and underneath your fingernails for at least 20 seconds.

4. Rinse thoroughly with warm water.

5. Dry your hands on a paper towel (not your shirt). Don't throw the paper towel away yet . . .

6. Open the bathroom door with the paper towel, so you don't touch that dirty handle. Prop the door open with your foot and toss the paper towel in the trash. (It's a good way to work on your basketball shot.)

What if you're nowhere near a sink but you need to clean your hands? You might want to carry around a container of liquid hand sanitizer (the kind that you squirt onto your hands and don't have to rinse off). Or you can use sanitizing wipes, which come in handy packets. Keep these products in your backpack, locker, purse, or pocket.

Here's a little reminder about *when* to wash your hands, in case your memory's fuzzy:

> # Fact!
>
> Before napkins came along, people wiped their hands and face right on the tablecloth.

* **BEFORE YOU EAT ANYTHING.** (Who wants to eat germs?)

* **AFTER YOU USE THE RESTROOM.** (Remember, there may be fecal matter hanging around on surfaces.)

* **BEFORE YOU HELP PREPARE FOOD.** (Your family isn't counting on eating germs from your hands.)

* **AFTER YOU TOUCH RAW MEAT.** (Those germs can be pretty dangerous.)

* **BEFORE YOU TOUCH A BABY.** (Babies have weaker immune systems and can't fight germs as easily.)

* **AFTER YOU PET YOUR DOG, CAT, REPTILE, OR FISH.** (Well, maybe you don't pet your fish, but you probably change its water.)

* **AFTER YOU CLEAN UP YOUR CAT'S LITTER BOX OR HOLD YOUR CAT.** (Cats may seem tidy, but remember they cover up their waste using their feet.)

* **AFTER YOUR DOG LICKS YOU.** (You never know where your dog's mouth has been: in the garbage, in the yard eating dead worms.)

* **AFTER PLAYING SPORTS OR VIDEO GAMES.** (Those joysticks can get pretty nasty.)

⭐ **WHEN YOU HOLD HANDS WITH SOMEONE.** (That person may like you, but they don't need your germs.)

⭐ **WHEN YOU'RE IN A RESTAURANT OR FAST-FOOD PLACE, ESPECIALLY IF YOU'RE ORDERING HAMBURGERS, TACOS, OR FRENCH FRIES.** (Those foods are a lot more appetizing if you eat them without a topping of nasty germs from your hands.)

⭐ **AFTER YOU COUGH OR SNEEZE.** (Think of all the germs your hand just caught. You can cough or sneeze into your sleeve to keep your hands free of the germs.)

⭐ **AFTER BLOWING YOUR NOSE.** (A tissue only holds so much.)

# WARTS, SWEATY PALMS, AND MORE

You've heard of warts. You may think of them as something on the end of a witch's nose or covering a warthog. But warts are a very human problem. Many people have warts on their hands or feet. If you have a wart on your hand, you'll see a raised bump with a rough surface and tiny black specks (which are the blood vessels).

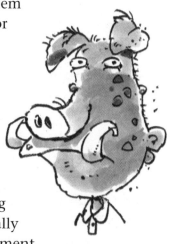

Warts are the most common skin infection you can get. In fact, there are more than 40 different types of warts. They're caused by touching viruses—not by touching frogs. Warts don't usually hurt, and they often disappear without any treatment.

However, you can buy an over-the-counter "acid" treatment to get rid of a wart. Another option is for a doctor to freeze it off or use an electric instrument to burn it off. Before trying any of these methods, you may just want to wait it out. The wart probably won't stick around for long.

Some people think warts are embarrassing. They wonder if other people will think they're dirty or gross for having a wart. You can tell people it's just a minor skin infection. Use an adhesive bandage to hide the wart temporarily, if you'd like. Some wart-removal products now include adhesive bandages that cover the wart until it's gone.

Another embarrassing hand problem is sweaty palms. Your palms are filled with sweat glands, so it would be highly unusual if you *didn't* have sweaty palms once in a while. But at your age, you may notice more sweat on your palms than you've had before. That's normal for kids approaching or going through puberty. Your sweat glands may go into "overdrive" just like your hormones.

Your emotions can trigger sweaty hands. If you're nervous, anxious, or stressed out (and who isn't some of the time?), your palms may start to sweat. This can be embarrassing if you're trying to hold hands with someone or if you have to shake hands with a person you're meeting for the first time. Instead of worrying about it too much—which can make your palms even wetter—tell yourself that everyone experiences sweaty palms sometimes. You're not the only one.

If sweaty palms are a real problem for you, try using an unscented antiperspirant that contains an ingredient called aluminum. Put the antiperspirant directly on your palms to help hold back the "waterworks."

You may have the opposite problem: dry, flaky, chapped hands. This condition tends to happen in winter because cold and windy weather dries out the natural skin oil and the moisture in your hands. You can use a moisturizing lotion that's made for dry hands. Apply it as often as needed, especially before bed so the lotion can soak in overnight.

As you now know, washing your hands is important. But a lot of hand washing can dry out already-dry hands. The best remedy is to leave your hands slightly damp after you wash them and apply some lotion. The lotion will help seal in the extra moisture.

Fact!

Thomas Jefferson started the custom of shaking hands instead of bowing.

★

Your palm has more than 2,000 sweat glands in an area about the size of a postage stamp.

"I hate it when my hands sweat. Some people wave their hands when they're sweaty to help dry them." —Huy, 12

# FINGERNAIL FACTS

Germs love to hide under your fingernails—just one more reason to wash your hands thoroughly. Knowing that there are germs under there might make you think twice the next time you feel like biting your nails.

Many of us don't pay attention to our fingernails until we have to cut them or we accidentally hit one of our nails with a hard object, like a hammer. When that happens, the tip of your finger hurts like crazy—but not as much as it would if you didn't have a nail protecting it. Fingernails not only protect your fingertips but also help you do everyday things like picking up a paperclip or coin, or separating a slice out of a pack of cheese.

Fingernails (and toenails) are made up of keratin, which is also a main ingredient in hair, claws, feathers, and animal horns. There are several parts to each nail. The *nail plate* is the part you trim; it isn't made up of any living tissue. The *cuticle* is a fold of skin at the base of the nail plate. It connects the nail plate to the skin and helps keeps infection away. The *nail bed* is the soft tissue under the nail plate; it contains lots of blood vessels and nerves.

Your fingernails grow constantly—about one-quarter inch per month. They may grow more quickly in warm weather than in cold. The nails on the hand you use most often tend to grow faster than the ones on your other hand.

How would you classify your nail-care habits? Do you fall into one of the following categories?

1. **NEAT AND CLEAN:** You clean your nails when you wash your hands, and you trim your nails when they get too long.

2. **NAIL-CONSCIOUS:** You think of your nails as an asset, like shiny, well-groomed hair.

3.  **FORGETFUL:** You remember how your nails look only if you've been biting them.

4.  **COULDN'T CARE LESS:** You come to school with ragged nails that are encrusted with dirt. (Just think of all the bacteria and skin flakes hanging around under there, keeping the dirt company.)

It's up to you to decide how much effort to put into your nails. If you tend to forget about your nails or ignore them altogether, it's time to put a bit more effort into caring for them. On the other hand, if you love your nails so much that you avoid certain sports or activities that might "ruin" them, you may want to consider a simpler nail-care routine. The best bet is to keep nails clean and neat.

To neaten up your nails, trim and file them as often as needed. You can buy nail-care tools such as a clipper and a nail file. You also can get an emery board, which is like a long, thin strip of cardboard with a sandpapery finish on both sides; this tool is used for filing and smoothing the nails. When you take a bath and your nails are soft, gently push back the cuticles using a file. You can buy products such as nail hardeners or strengtheners, if needed.

Some girls enjoy using nail polish. It's fun to experiment with different colors and looks. If you're into dark colors like black, protect your nails from staining by applying a clear base coat first.

If you want to try fake fingernails, be aware of the problems they can cause. Fake fingernails that are glued over your real nails shut off the oxygen supply to

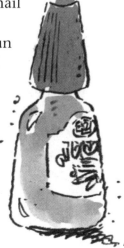

## Fact!

In the year 2000, a man from India, who holds the Guinness World Record for the longest fingernails, finally clipped them. He said the nails, which were 4 feet long, were causing him pain in his left wrist and arm.

★

In 4000 B.C., Egyptians painted their fingernails by dipping their fingers into henna, the plant dye they also used to color their hair.

your nail beds. Sometimes, infections start underneath. Temporary press-on fake nails may be a better option because you can remove them after a few days.

Remember that, although your fingernails may seem pretty hard, they're actually porous. This means they have tiny holes or pores that can absorb liquids. So if you spend a lot of time in a chlorinated pool, for example, you may notice weakened fingernails. You can put some petroleum jelly on them to protect them. Petroleum jelly also can help lubricate dry, brittle nails.

## Nail Problems

Are you a nail biter or chewer? If you are, you know these are hard habits to break. You may bite or chew your nails when you are stressed out, tense, or bored.

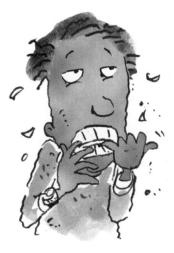

Some people only nibble— others chew their nails down to the nail bed. This takes away the nails' ability to protect the fingertips. Plus, it leaves the nails looking ragged and torn.

If you want to stop the nail-biting habit, you can do it! Try thinking about all the germs you're putting into your mouth when you chew. It may also help to keep your nails filed smooth—the fewer rough edges to tempt you, the better. Another option is to buy a product that's designed to prevent nail biting (the bitter taste supposedly stops you from chewing).

Be aware of what triggers your nail biting. Homework? Tests? A big game? During those times, make a conscious effort to keep your fingers away from your mouth and figure out some healthier ways to deal with stress.

Another common problem is hangnails, which means that a bit of skin has separated from the cuticle. Hangnails are painful and may even bleed. It's tempting to pick at or bite hangnails, which usually worsens the problem. Instead, take a small pair of scissors and *gently* trim the loose skin. Don't go any deeper than you need to in order to cut the hangnail. Afterward, put some first-aid ointment on your finger and cover the spot with an adhesive bandage. Then leave it alone until it has healed.

If your nails are yellow, you may have a nail fungus. (Dark nail polish and tar from cigarettes may turn the nails yellow as well.) Another symptom of fungus is separation of the nail from the nail bed. If you have this problem, see a doctor for treatment. It won't go away on its own.

★ ★ ★

Thanks to your hands and fingers, you can play a piano piece, swing a baseball bat, write a poem, and pet a dog. Think of all the other wonderful things your hands can do. Aren't they worth taking care of and protecting? All in favor, raise your hands!

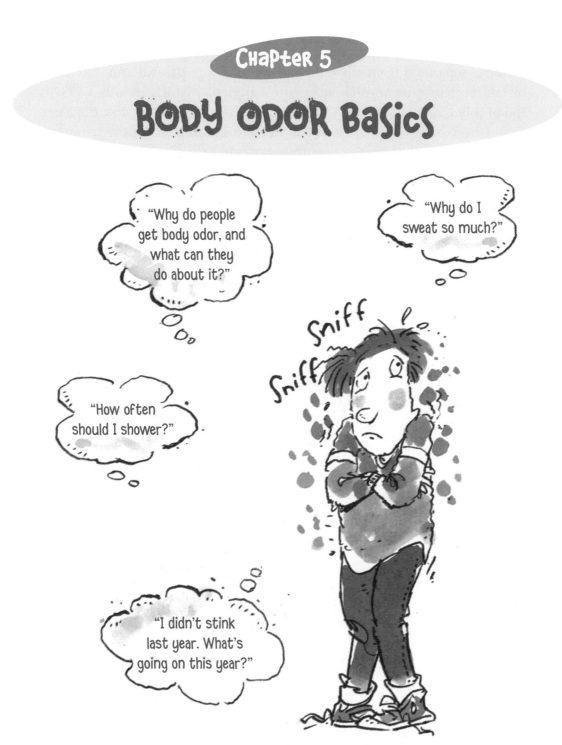

**E**ek! What reeks? It's probably your body odor—or somebody else's.

Lately, you may have noticed a certain scent wafting through your classroom or in the locker room. By afternoon, the air may be ripe with unpleasant smells. Perhaps your teacher has started placing air fresheners in different parts of the room. What's this all about? Puberty.

During puberty, your body matures. Along with that, your sweat glands start to work harder than they did when you were younger. Those hardworking sweat glands produce some funky odors. Although these odors are natural, they may not be too pleasant. But don't sweat it—staying fresh and smelling clean during puberty *is* possible. This chapter will tell you how.

## SWEAT: A LIFESAVER

Just like other parts of your body, your sweat glands have a job to do. They're supposed to keep you from overheating. Without them, you'd be in big trouble.

Suppose you're at soccer practice on a scorching, humid day. You and your teammates run through drills, sprinting up and down the field. You gulp water every chance you get and you're perspiring, or sweating, like crazy.

Sweat is the salty liquid that seeps from millions of sweat glands located all over your body. Sweat itself is 99 percent water and 1 percent other ingredients such as sodium (salt), chloride, potassium, urea (found in urine), ammonia, uric acid, and phosphorus. When your body releases sweat through your pores, your skin cools down.

Your normal body temperature is about 98.6 degrees. Sweating helps keep you close to this temperature, even when it's hot outside. Think of your sweat glands as your personal cooling system. Have you ever seen a car conked out on the side of the road, with steam pouring from its

### Fact!

Most of your sweat glands are located on the palms of your hands and soles of your feet.

★

People in hot climates often enjoy spicy foods that kick their sweat glands into gear and help cool them off.

"When you think about sweating, you sweat even more!"
—Colin, 1o

hood? You don't want to overheat like that. You can thank your sweat glands for being on the job day and night, keeping you cool.

If you look around, you might notice that some people seem to stay much drier than others. People sweat differently. Some seem to perspire heavily while doing everyday things like sitting in class. Others seem to sweat mostly when working out.

No matter what your sweat level may be, you might feel a bit uncomfortable. It's no fun, for example, to run around getting soaked with sweat during gym, and then return to a hot classroom. As you listen to your teacher, you may feel sweat pouring from your armpits and wonder who turned on the sprinklers.

If you're sweating more than usual, it's most likely a result of puberty—and it's totally normal. However, some people have a rare condition called *hyperhydrosis*, which causes them to sweat heavily under the arms, on their palms, or on the soles of their feet. Heavy sweating can be embarrassing, so if this is happening to you, talk to a doctor. The condition can be treated with special products or medications, depending on how severe the problem is.

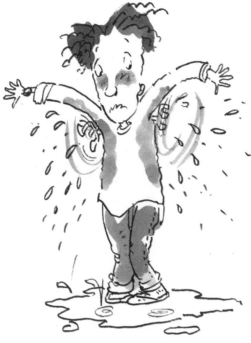

## Say Hello to B.O.

When you think of sweat, you might think of body odor, otherwise known as "B.O." Although the two are connected, there's more to the story. Sweat actually is odorless when it leaves your pores. Remember all that bacteria swarming over your body? (See page 25 for more about that.) Bacteria love a warm, moist environment such as a sweaty armpit. The bacteria react with the sweat and release odors.

You have two kinds of sweat glands: *eccrine* and *apocrine*. Most of your sweat comes from your 2 million eccrine sweat glands, which are located in areas like your hands, feet, and forehead. Those glands create the type of sweat you get in your palms when you play video games or when you have to give a speech. Sometimes, you have to wipe the sweat out of your eyes when you're playing basketball or riding your skateboard. It's annoying when these areas drip with sweat, but at least they don't smell. You probably don't get stinky hands or a rank forehead.

The apocrine sweat glands, on the other hand, kick into gear as you go through puberty. These glands are located in your armpits, around your nipples, and in your groin area. Apocrine glands produce thicker sweat that has an odor. When bacteria mix with this sweat, more stinky fumes are created—and before you know it, B.O. has come to call.

Sweat and bacteria aren't the only culprits when it comes to B.O. Sebum (skin oil) plays a part as well. Take a moment to rub your finger alongside your nose; you'll see some shiny oil on your finger when you're done. That's sebum, or the oil that protects your skin and hair.

While it's easy to notice if you have an oily nose, you might not be aware of the skin oil produced on other parts of your body, like under your arms. The sebum is all over your skin on different body parts, though. (Good thing, too, or we'd all look as dry as crocodiles.)

The drawback is that the oil can get as stale and funky-smelling as spoiled cooking grease. Plus, the oil is a trap for dirt, dead skin cells, bacteria, and apocrine sweat. This mixture can create quite a stink. Fortunately, good old soap and water will wash it all away.

## Fact!

Bacteria are so tiny that a dozen of them could line up across just one of your pores.

★

Caffeine, which is found in sodas and coffee, can stimulate sweat glands and encourage body odor. Strong smelling foods like onions and garlic can add to body odor, too.

"The first time my friend found out she had body odor was really funny. She was sitting on her grandmother's lap, and her grandmother said, 'Dang, don't you use deodorant?'"
—Laura, 12

At your age, you probably need to take a shower or bath every day. Washing yourself daily removes dirt and sweat, kills germs, and helps you avoid body odor.

## Keeping B.O. at Bay

Here's a question worthy of debate: Which is better, showers or baths? The "Shower Team" might say that showers are quicker and cleaner (since you're not sitting in your own dirt). But the "Bath Team" may counter that nothing's more relaxing than a good, long soak in the tub. Both sides make a good point.

The key is to wash *every* day, whether in the shower or the bath. This is especially important during hotter months, when you sweat more. If you have dry, itchy skin, you may not want to spend too much time in hot water, because it can dry out your skin more. Take shorter baths or showers, in cooler water, and follow up with a moisturizer.

If bathing or showering sometimes isn't possible, you still have options. You can wash your underarms in the sink, using a washcloth or a wet paper towel. Drugstores sell disposable towelettes that contain soap; all you have to do is wipe away the dirt and sweat, and then toss the towelette in the trash afterward.

Getting the sweat and oil off your body, even temporarily, helps you win the body odor battle.

You may wonder what type of soap to use on your skin when you wash. There are lots of brands to choose from. Have you ever been to one of those bath shops where they make soap from every ingredient imaginable? Does anybody *really* need soap made from walnut shells or avocado pits? Fancy, expensive soaps aren't any better than the kinds you find on the drugstore shelves. You don't have to spend a bundle to get clean.

# A SHORT HISTORY OF SOAP

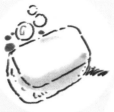

No one knows for sure, but legend says that soap was discovered by accident when ancient Romans sacrificed animals to their gods. Rain fell, mixing with the animal fat and the ashes from fires. The mixture was carried into the soil. Women found that when this clay soil got onto clothes they were washing, it made them cleaner.

A crude type of soap was made in the second century in France, and soap making was an established craft by the seventh century in Italy and Spain. Until the eighteenth century, people mainly used soap for washing clothes.

In 1791, a French chemist discovered a way to make soda ash from common salt, and people learned they could make their own soap cheaply at home. Before then, only rich people could afford soap.

To make soap at home, American women collected animal fat and cooking grease, as well as wood ashes from their fireplaces. They poured hot water through the ashes and mixed it with the boiled fat. The result was a harsh lye soap.

Around 1850, soap makers began to produce soap for mass consumption. People known as "soap boilers" bought fat from families, made the fat into soap, and sold it back to the families.

Today, there are many types of soaps to choose from, but most are still made from fats.

Any type of soap will lift sebum, dirt, and bacteria off your skin. (For more information about different types of soaps and cleansers, see pages 26–27.) You may have to experiment with several brands until you find a soap or body cleanser with a scent and price you like. Each time you shower or bathe, be sure to thoroughly wash your armpits and groin area.

Deodorant soaps and antibacterial soaps can help fight B.O. Deodorant soaps contain special ingredients to neutralize odor. Antibacterial soaps are designed to kill bacteria. These products help keep

"I play sports, and there isn't much you can do to solve B.O. The only things that help are taking showers after games and wearing deodorant. I had times when I smelled really bad after a game, but everyone else smelled bad, too."
—Ashley, 13

odor away, but remember that your body constantly produces more sweat, oil, and odors. Soap can only work for so long.

## THE "DISH" ON DEODORANT

Antiperspirants and deodorants came on the scene in the 1890s. But it wasn't until the 1940s that Americans got into these products in a big way. At the time, people enjoyed listening to radio "soap operas," which were sponsored by soap companies. Suddenly, people started buying a lot more soap. They believed the message advertisers were selling—that being clean and smelling fresh was important.

Today, advertisers are still selling this message, and not just to adults. Companies that sell cosmetics are advertising to preteens and teens more than ever before. You've probably seen lots of magazine ads or TV commercials telling you how important it is to never sweat or smell. (You'd have to be a robot not to!) That's how these companies get your money. They want you to feel self-conscious about how your body smells. The more products you buy, the more money the cosmetic companies make.

Keep in mind that people around the world have different attitudes about personal hygiene. Most Americans today think body odor is a total turnoff. They tend to back away from someone who smells a bit "ripe." In other countries around the world, people consider sweat to be perfectly natural. They don't mind the odors as much. And in some parts of the world, people never use underarm deodorant at all.

Go to any drugstore in America, however, and you're likely to find a bunch of deodorants and antiperspirants to choose from. Some stores have entire *aisles* devoted to these products. For some reason, people in the United States think B.O. should be avoided at all costs.

What's the difference between deodorants and antiperspirants anyway? Deodorants are supposed to get rid of odor; they have special ingredients that kill bacteria. Antiperspirants, on the other hand, work to keep you dry. They contain aluminum salts to clog the pores in your underarms so the sweat won't come out. Some antiperspirants may have bacteria-killing chemicals, too. You also can find combination deodorant/antiperspirants that are designed to fight odor and wetness. These underarm products come in sticks, roll-ons, sprays, gels, and creams. Try out a few to find one you like.

Be aware that companies selling these items want to convince you that their product will help you be more "feminine," more "macho," or more like a teen. But most of these products contain the exact same ingredients. The only difference may be in the packaging, the price, or the perfumes that are used.

Follow the directions on the product so you don't use too much or too little. If you're trying a roll-on, apply a thin, even layer under your arms and let it dry before you get dressed. If you prefer a spray, use only about a two-second shot under your arms. If you use a solid, watch out for white stains on your clothes—this might signal that you've put on too much of the product.

Maybe you want to try natural odor-fighting products that don't contain as many chemical ingredients. Look for these items in natural foods stores. Many of these products use bacteria-fighting herbs like chamomile, rosemary, and extracts of green tea. You might want to try a deodorant stone made of crystals that contain bacteria-fighting mineral salts. It may seem strange to rub a deodorant stone under your arm, but many people have found that the stones are longer-lasting and cheaper than other deodorants. For an inexpensive homemade antiperspirant, apply a few drops of witch hazel with a cotton ball.

Fact!

Deodorants are considered to be "cosmetics" because they work on the skin's surface. But antiperspirants are called over-the-counter drugs because they change how the body functions.

"Once, I didn't put on deodorant, and the guy I had a crush on said something to me about it."
—Macey, 12

What if you still notice an odor after using products designed to keep you smelling fresh? Maybe you didn't cover the entire underarm area, or perhaps the product has simply worn off. You may need to reapply a fresh coat.

If you think you're not staying dry enough, you may need to apply an antiperspirant twice a day—in the morning and at bedtime. Using the product before you go to bed will allow the ingredients to absorb into your skin while you're less active. (Take your shower the night before, too, so the antiperspirant isn't washed away the next morning.) It's helpful to apply the product on dry skin, so wait a bit to cool off if you've just bathed or worked out. In addition, you could dust your underarms with an absorbent powder or talc. Baking soda or cornstarch straight from the kitchen cupboard might work well, too.

Now that you know so much about deodorants and antiperspirants, staying fresh may not be a problem for you. But it may be a problem for someone you know. Perhaps you have a friend who has B.O. and you're not sure how to break the news.

It's hard to tell a friend or classmate that he or she has body odor, but if you do it in a friendly, supportive way, that person will probably thank you. Be sure to keep the conversation private so no one else hears. Don't come on too strong and say something like, "Hey, you really stink! Why don't you do something about it?" Instead, you might say, "I noticed that your deodorant isn't working as well as it should. I've tried a brand that really works. You may want to try it, too." You could add that everyone smells sometimes, and it's no big deal. If you don't feel comfortable telling the person face-to-face, you could send a friendly but anonymous letter.

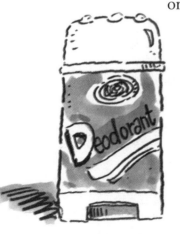

# HOW FRESH ARE YOUR CLOTHES?

Have you ever showered, put on a clean shirt, and headed off to school—only to notice a little too late that the shirt isn't as fresh as the rest of you? Your body may have been clean and fresh, but your clothes told a different story.

The armpits of your favorite shirts—the ones you wear most often—may have residue from sweat and deodorant. Sometimes, you'll even notice a yellow color on the underarms of your light-colored shirts. Certain brands of detergent may be able remove these stains and odors, but not always. Give your shirts the "sniff test" to see if they've really gotten clean.

You're probably aware that it's not a great idea to raid the dirty clothes hamper when you're getting dressed. If you thought the clothes were dirty enough to put there, they need to stay there until laundry day. Take the time to search for something clean to wear instead. It may be tempting to try to get one last wearing out of your coolest shirt, but how cool will you feel in a dirty, smelly, wrinkly shirt?

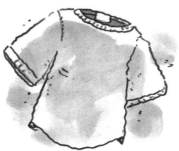

Remember, the apocrine sweat glands around your armpits, nipples, and groin area have become more active. It's important to keep the clothing that touches those areas as clean as possible. Wash your shirts, bras, and underwear regularly. And always put on a clean pair of underwear in the morning. You'll feel and smell much fresher if you follow this advice.

✦ ✦ ✦

Now you know how to arm those underarms! With the right tools, you can keep yourself fresher and drier, even on the hottest days. Be glad that you sweat. It's your body's way of staying cool.

## Fact!

Medieval families washed their clothes in soap made from wood ash and scraps of meat fat. Even worse, they added old urine to it for "bleach"!

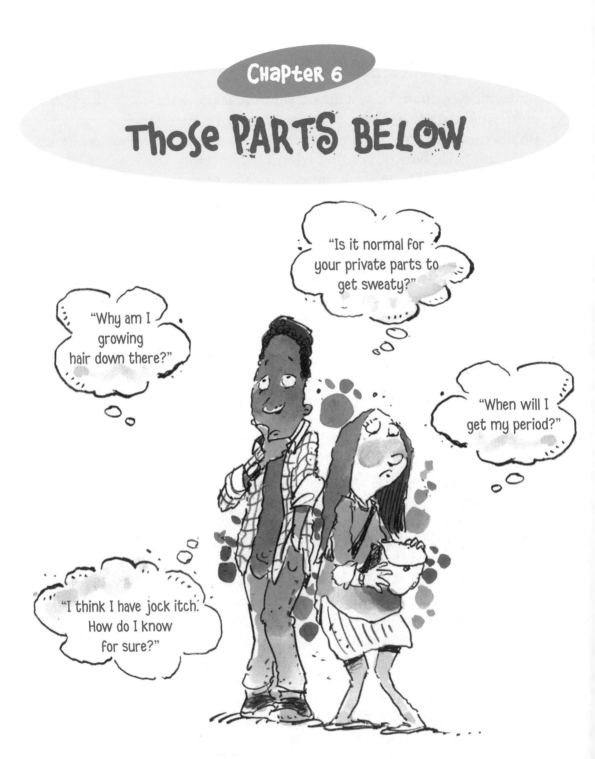

**O**ur culture has a weird view of people's groins, or private parts. On the one hand we don't talk openly about what's going on. (We call it private.) On the other hand, ads on television and in magazines tell us we have to deodorize these areas, especially if we're girls. At your age, things are changing down there, inside and out. Here's some information to help you know what to expect.

## WHAT'S GOING ON DOWN THERE?

Most of you reading this book are at an age where you're noticing lots of body changes. Keep in mind that you're becoming an adult, and the process takes a long time. Everyone gets there on different schedules. If your friends are undergoing physical changes ahead of you, don't worry about it too much. You'll get there eventually. Your growth is probably similar to that of your parents, so ask them about their experiences.

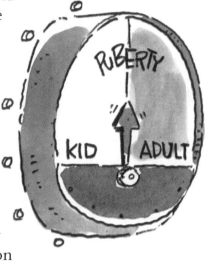

Maybe you have the opposite problem: you seem to be getting there too fast. You may notice changes happening to you that aren't happening to other people yet. This is normal, too. Soon enough, other people will catch up and you won't feel so alone.

Some of the changes that happen aren't even noticeable to others, because they take place internally (inside you). For example, it's not obvious to others that your ovaries are growing, or that you're producing sperm. Most likely, you'll learn about changes like these in health class at school, in talks with a parent or another adult, or by reading more about puberty. You can find books about the topic in any library, or you can look at Web sites that deal with puberty and other body changes.

Briefly, some of the developments for girls include the following:

★ the hips get wider

★ straight, fine pubic hair appears

★ the vagina gets bigger

★ pubic hair grows darker and coarser

★ the ovaries become larger

★ menstruation (your period) starts

Boys typically experience the changes of puberty later than girls do. Some of the developments for boys include the following:

★ the testicles and scrotum get bigger

★ the scrotum becomes redder, and the texture changes

★ fine pubic hair appears, and it eventually gets darker and thicker

★ the penis grows in length and width, and its skin darkens

★ the first ejaculation, or release of semen from the penis, occurs

None of these changes happen overnight, so you'll have time to get used to them. Sometimes, the changes are uncomfortable; other times, they're actually a bit exciting. Although the changes may be embarrassing to talk about, it helps to discuss them with a friend or parent.

## Those Parts Below (Boys)

Boys and girls have different "equipment." So it makes sense to talk about the different issues separately. This section is for boys, but girls can read it, too. On pages 87–89, you'll find information about girls' parts (boys can read that section as well).

Any discussion of boys' parts has to start with the penis. After all, this sexual organ is a pretty important body part. Penis size can vary a lot from boy to boy. If you're worried about your penis size, you're not the only one. This is a big source of anxiety for many boys. Whether or not you have a big penis makes little difference in how the organ actually works.

The penis is designed to respond to stimulation, like when you touch it or when you're thinking about sex. Blood rushes into the area, and the penis swells and gets hard (this is called an erection). The surge of hormones during puberty means you might have lots of erections, even when you don't want them—like during school. Erections are totally normal but may be embarrassing. You can wear long shirts or carry a notebook to use as a "shield."

Some boys have their penis *circumcised* at birth, which means the foreskin that covers the head of the penis is surgically removed. Parents have this optional procedure done for religious or cultural reasons. Circumcised and uncircumcised penises look different when they're soft. You can see the head or *glans* of a circumcised penis, but the glans is covered by foreskin on an uncircumcised one.

Keeping the penis clean is important, whether it's circumcised or uncircumcised. Wash your genital area every day, in a shower or bath. You can use a deodorant or an antibacterial soap, if you'd like (for more on soaps, see pages 26–27). If you're uncircumcised, you'll need to pull back the foreskin to wash out the glans area. Pull it back only as far as is comfortable.

Many boys notice small bumps on their penis and wonder if the bumps are normal. Most likely, they're just pimples or blackheads. Or they might be *pearly penile papules,* a strange name for harmless, flesh-colored bumps on the head of the penis. About 15 percent of teen boys get them during puberty. Symptoms like warts, blisters, or painful places on your genitals indicate a more serious problem and mean you need to see a doctor.

Many boys, and men, too, are prone to getting a rash known as *jock itch.* If you've had jock itch, you might vividly remember an itching, burning sensation in your groin. (It's hard to ignore a feeling that makes you want to scratch your privates.) If you work out or play sports and you use locker rooms or public showers, you're a prime candidate for this irritation, which is caused by a fungus.

"I remember when I was in seventh grade, and it seemed like I had erections all the time! I'd walk around with my books in front of my lap."
—Anonymous, 14

"I'm embarrassed because my penis is little."
—Andy, 9

If you think you've got jock itch, look for a red rash and itching around your scrotum, anus, and inner thighs. You can treat this condition by keeping the area clean and dry, and by washing only with mild soaps. (Harsh soaps will aggravate the rash.) You can apply over-the-counter creams or powders made to treat jock itch. Sometimes, it helps to wear looser-fitting clothing, too. Wash your sporting clothes often to get rid of the fungus and change your underwear frequently, including your jockstrap.

If you're wondering what a jockstrap is, it's an elastic supporter that pulls your testicles up close to your body. Because your sexual organs are on the outside of your body, they're more easily injured, especially when playing sports like football. When playing rough contact sports, you can wear an athletic cup inside your jock strap for even more protection. Jockstraps are sold according to waist size not penis size—so don't feel embarrassed picking up a package marked "small."

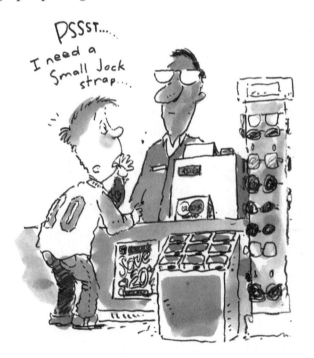

In movies and on TV shows, it's supposed to be funny when a guy gets kicked or kneed in the "balls" (testicles). If you've had this happen, you probably weren't laughing. It hurts so much you can get sick to your stomach. That's why wearing a cup or supporter during sports is a good idea.

## Those Parts Below (Girls)

If you're a girl, the changes happening down there may seem like a big mystery because most of them take place inside. The most noticeable change on the outside may be the growth of pubic hair (you can read more about that on pages 91–92).

However, girls have one big event that signals puberty, and this is, of course, menstruation. Getting your period is the sign that your body is able to make a baby. That's very different than being READY to make a baby. You're not mature enough for such a huge responsibility.

At your age, you may not have started your period yet. Be patient; it will happen eventually. Whether you have your period or not, you've probably got lots of questions about what it's like. Talk with your mom, your older sister, your aunt, or another female adult you trust. They've been through it and can give you some good information.

Usually, before a girl starts her period, she may notice a small amount of fluid, called discharge, from her vagina. This normal discharge is usually clear or slightly white in color. Vaginal discharge is your body's way of cleaning itself of bacteria, old cells, and mucus.

Sometimes, discharge can be a sign of infection. If you notice other symptoms, such as irritated skin, itching, or a bad odor, you may have an infection. You'll need to see a doctor to find out. Although itchiness can signal an infection, it simply may be a reaction to soaps, perfumes, or detergents. Switch to a milder soap and avoid deodorant sprays down there. You also may need to ask your dad or mom to buy perfume-free laundry detergent.

To prevent vaginal infections, wash your genitals thoroughly every day. Wear cotton underpants, because cotton allows your skin to "breathe." Avoid using products that contain talc or wearing tight clothing. Also, be sure to change out of sweaty underwear or a wet swimsuit as quickly as possible. Experts believe that infections can be transmitted

A popular fad on college campuses in the 1960s was for men to make "panty raids" on women's dormitories to take their underpants.

★

Women have probably used tampons for thousands of years, but the first commercial production of tampons in the United States began in the late 1920s or early 1930s.

"Periods are just a normal thing all girls go through in their lives. You don't have to be scared of them."
—Morgan, 12

when using someone else's dirty towel, washcloth, or wet bathing suit, so don't use other people's belongings.

Regardless of the messages you get from ads in magazines and on television, you don't need to use special sprays and powders to keep your genital area clean—even when you have your period. The vagina is a self-cleaning organ. All you need to do is wash the outside parts each day. Ignore those ads telling you to use a "second" deodorant (besides the one for your armpits). In fact, these sprays have been known to cause allergic reactions or even infections because they're loaded with perfume. Many girls and women worry about whether they smell clean. The truth is, all women have a natural vaginal scent, and it doesn't smell bad.

On the other hand, on days when you have your period, you may not feel as clean. When menstrual blood hits the air, bacteria begins to collect. The bacteria can cause odors. You may want to wash more often on those days, but it's not absolutely necessary. If you change your menstrual pads or tampons regularly (at least every three to four hours), odor shouldn't be a huge problem.

Speaking of tampons and pads, you may wonder how they work and which product is best for you. Most girls start out using pads because they're easy. You pull the adhesive strip, stick the pad in your underwear, and you're done.

Tampons are inserted inside the vagina, which is a little trickier to do until you get the hang of it. You can practice with smaller-sized tampons at first—even before you start your period. Just follow the instructions that come with the tampons. It takes a little practice, but you'll eventually get comfortable with using tampons. You can choose "deodorant" tampons, if you want, but they aren't necessary; you may have a reaction to the perfumes they contain. Keeping yourself washed should be enough.

Once you start menstruating, you may worry that everyone in the world will know. But they'll only know if you tell them. If you want to talk about your period, don't feel shy about it. Periods happen to every girl at some point. You also can discuss any concerns you may have with an adult you trust. Look at books about getting your period or go online to check out Web sites that deal with the topic. These are great ways to get answers to all your questions.

# TIPS FOR BEING PREPARED FOR YOUR PERIOD

★ Keep extra underwear and pads or tampons in your locker.

★ Wear dark clothes if you're expecting your period and you're worried about leaks.

★ Wear panty liners (very thin pads) to protect your underwear, if you'd like.

★ Carry pads or tampons with you. Some are folded into tiny packages so you can hide them in your backpack or binder.

★ Ask your mom or dad about pain relievers you can take for premenstrual syndrome (PMS). Pain relievers can help you with the discomforts of cramping, headaches, or fatigue.

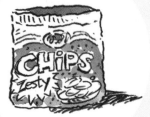

★ Be aware of the links between consuming caffeine and salt and getting a worse case of PMS. You may want to cut back on the soda and cheese puffs during that time of the month.

## OTHER "DOWN THERE" ISSUES

Why do people have pubic hair? Why do they wear underwear? Good questions.

The answers aren't easy, though.

If you think back to Chapter 5, "Body Odor Basics," you might remember that there are two types of sweat glands, *eccrine* and *apocrine*. The apocrine glands, located in your underarms, around your nipples, and in your groin area, are the ones that lead to stinky smells (when the sweat combines with bacteria). In your groin area, the apocrine glands are located around your genitals and anus.

If you recall a time when you were hot and sweaty, you might remember that your underwear got wet, too. That's the result of your apocrine sweat glands doing their job. It's helpful to have on a pair of underwear to absorb the sweat and odors, and help protect the tender skin in those areas. In other words, wearing underwear is practical. That may be the best reason for their use.

There's no doubt, however, that historically underwear was worn for other reasons—the main one being modesty. Throughout the ages, people have been shy about their bodies, especially the genital area. In the 1800s, men wore union suits, or pairs of underwear that snugly covered their bodies from their ankles to their neck. During the same time period, women's undergarments included corsets made of whale bone to tighten their waistline, plus pantaloons and slips. Today, our choices for underwear are much simpler (lucky for us).

Whether you choose fancy underpants or basic briefs, make sure they're made of cotton, a breathable fabric. And change your underwear every day. After you shower or bathe, put on fresh "undies" to stay cleaner and prevent odors. If you need to change your underwear more often than once a day, that's okay. Puberty leads to

increased sweating and hormonal changes, and sometimes not-so-fresh underwear. You may have extra laundry, but that isn't a big deal.

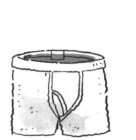
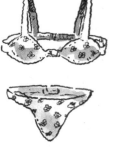

Fact!

When women
wore two-piece
swimsuits in the
1940s, everyone was
shocked. Actually,
bikinis have been
found in paintings
from the 4th cen-
tury in Sicily.

No one really knows for sure why we have pubic hair.
Some people believe it was originally for the purpose of
keeping our genitals warm. Other people think girls and
women have pubic hair to protect the vagina from dirt (in
the same way nose hairs protect the nose). But then, why
do boys and men have pubic hair?

Some people think pubic hair may be nature's way of
saying, "Yoo-hoo! Look at me! I'm sexually mature!" One
other theory is that pubic hair catches people's sexual
smells, which may attract a member of the opposite sex.

Whatever the reason, girls start seeing pubic hair
around age nine and boys around age ten. In both sexes,
the first pubic hairs are straight and fine in texture. They
later become curly and coarse. Pubic hair varies with each
person. Some people end up with thick, dark hair; others
have reddish or blond pubic hair. Some people have lots
of pubic hair, and some not so much.

Girls may have more of an issue with this patch of
hair than boys do. That's because, in many cultures, girls
are expected to have hair only on their head. Because
girls naturally grow hair on other parts of their body,
many are constantly in search of methods to get rid of
the furry stuff under their arms, on their upper lip, and

on their legs. The pubic area is no exception. Many girls hate it when they've got pubic hair sticking out of the edges of their swimsuit. This is called the *bikini line,* and for some girls, it requires constant attention during the summer.

There are several ways to keep that bikini line free of hair—all of which are temporary and *optional.* You can trim the hair with scissors to keep it neater. Or you can shave it, which will keep the hair away for a few days. You may get some stubble, irritation, or ingrown hairs, though. Ingrown hairs are little red bumps that get sore; they indicate that the hair has grown back into your skin.

Another hair-removal option is waxing, which requires painting warm wax on the area and ripping it off along with your hair. You also can try a depilatory, which contains chemicals to remove hair. Test a small area first to make sure products like these won't seriously irritate your skin.

## Toilet Etiquette

You may feel like we're going back to Potty Training 101, but let's talk about what's happening in the bathroom. Why? Because you may have questions you're afraid to ask anyone.

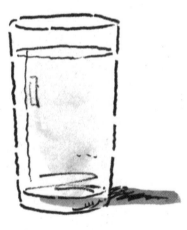

It's the job of your kidneys to filter waste from your blood and produce urine (pee). Urine is made up of these wastes, plus extra water and salts. People release about four to eight cups of urine every day. Next time you go to the bathroom, check to see what color your urine is. It should be light yellow to clear. If you don't drink enough water, it might be a dark gold color. Make sure you're drinking at least six to eight cups of water per day.

"I wet my bed one night, and I was so embarrassed to tell my mom. I thought I'd die of embarrassment!" "Just me,"—10

# BED-WETTING CAN HAPPEN TO ANYONE

About 1 in every 100 teens wets the bed. It's true! And it happens to twice as many guys as girls. What's the cause? Experts think bed-wetting happens to older kids who sleep so soundly that they don't wake up when they need to go. Some kids simply have grown faster than their bladder has. If you have this problem, take heart. You'll probably outgrow it in a few years. In the evening, avoid drinking lots of liquids after dinner—especially ones that contain caffeine. Above all, know that bed-wetting isn't your fault.

Now let's talk about what comes out the other end. You may have heard the term "bowel movements," which means feces, or poop. Feces are formed from what's left of your food after it's been digested, plus bacteria, dead cells, salts, and water. To help keep your feces soft, eat foods that contain lots of fiber (like fruits and vegetables). How often should you go? It differs from person to person. Some have bowel movements several times a day, while others go a few times a week.

You might see ads on television talking about "irregularity," meaning constipation. That's when your poop is hard and dry, and it's difficult for you to go. If you think you might be constipated, eat fiber and drink lots of water; exercise helps, too.

Sometimes, people take laxatives to help move things along, but these products aren't always safe for someone your age. You won't know when the laxative's going to kick in (like in the middle of playing basketball or while taking a test), so you're probably better off using a more natural remedy.

## Fact!

There are people around the world who drink urine as a healthy drink.

★

In the Middle Ages, people used chamber pots for toilets. These pots were like a bucket or bowl. With no way to flush, they simply dumped the contents out the windows and onto the street. Look out below!

★

When people travel to other countries, they often get diarrhea because they drink or eat different types of germs than they're used to. This traveler's diarrhea is sometimes called "Montezuma's revenge" or the "Aztec two-step."

Fact!

In the late 1800s, toilet paper was produced in U.S. factories. Many people were reluctant to buy it at first because they were using old newspapers, corn cobs, and catalogs quite cheaply.

★

Throughout history, people have used various items to wipe themselves, including twigs, grass, leaves, feathers, oyster shells, tree bark, newspapers, and sponges on sticks.

★

In Europe in the Middle Ages, urine was collected in big containers, and the ammonia in it was sold to help make leather goods.

Diarrhea is the opposite problem; it means your poop is runny, and you have to go frequently. Illness or stress can lead to diarrhea. Usually, diarrhea goes away in a couple of days. In the meantime, drink diluted juices, sports drinks, or broth to make up for the amount of water and salt you're losing. Tell your mom or dad so they can help find out what might have given you diarrhea.

When you wipe after urinating or having a bowel movement, take the time to clean yourself thoroughly. Urine and feces contain waste material, and are full of bacteria. You don't want this material hanging around on your skin any longer than necessary. Plus, wiping away the residue helps get rid of odor.

Wipe from front to back, especially if you're a girl. This wipes the bacteria away from your genital area and may prevent infections. Good old toilet paper is usually enough to do the job. Or you may decide to use wet cleansing wipes to clean yourself after using the bathroom.

Sometimes, you may feel a bit sore and itchy in your anal area. This could be a result of over-cleaning. When you wipe, be gentle—don't act like you're scrubbing a greasy pan. On the other hand, a sore bottom could mean you're not cleaning yourself well enough. Be sure to use enough toilet paper with each wipe.

Have you ever had someone use your bathroom, only to leave dribbles of pee or poop on the toilet seat? Talk about bad manners! Here are a few things to keep in mind when you use a toilet, whether it's yours or someone else's:

1. If you lift the seat up, put it down when you're done out of courtesy for the next user.

2. Shut the lid on the toilet before you flush. (There are millions of particles of pee and poop that fly into the air during each flush. If there's a toothbrush sitting nearby, guess where some of those particles land?)

3. If you accidentally mess up the toilet seat, wipe it up. (Other people will thank you for leaving a clean seat.)

4. If you use the final sheets of toilet paper, replace the roll. (It's a frustrating moment when you're sitting on the "throne," only to discover there's nothing to wipe with.)

Some kids don't like to use public restrooms and may "hold it" all day. This isn't good for your health. If you're worried about having a bowel movement in a public place, carry a small air freshener in your purse or backpack so you can get rid of the odor. If you're afraid to use a public toilet because it looks dirty, you could line the seat with toilet paper before sitting down. The chances of "catching" anything from a toilet seat are slim. You may catch some germs but nothing that won't wash away during your next shower or bath.

Fortunately, many public bathrooms in schools, libraries, and malls are relatively clean and useable. In some countries, this just isn't the case. World travelers can tell you about "squat" toilets that consist of a platform to squat on over a deep pit. On the other hand, public toilets in some areas of Japan are technological wonders. Exceptionally clean, they even have a button to push to add the sound of running water to cover up any "bathroom" sounds people may make!

★ ★ ★

Now you know more about what's happening "down there." It's not such a big mystery. The next time you feel embarrassed about something going on in that area, just remember that—somewhere, somehow—someone else is going through the same thing. Maybe you won't feel like talking about any of these private issues, but at least you'll know you're not alone!

Fact!

Most Americans use about 9 sheets of toilet paper each time they go to the bathroom, which adds up to about 57 sheets every day.

★

Males take an average of 45 seconds to use the bathroom, and females take about 79 seconds. That's why there's often a long line of girls and women waiting to use the restroom in public places.

"I went hunting with my dad and had to go to the bathroom in the woods. I didn't have toilet paper so I wiped with leaves that turned out to be poison ivy!"
—Anonymous, 12

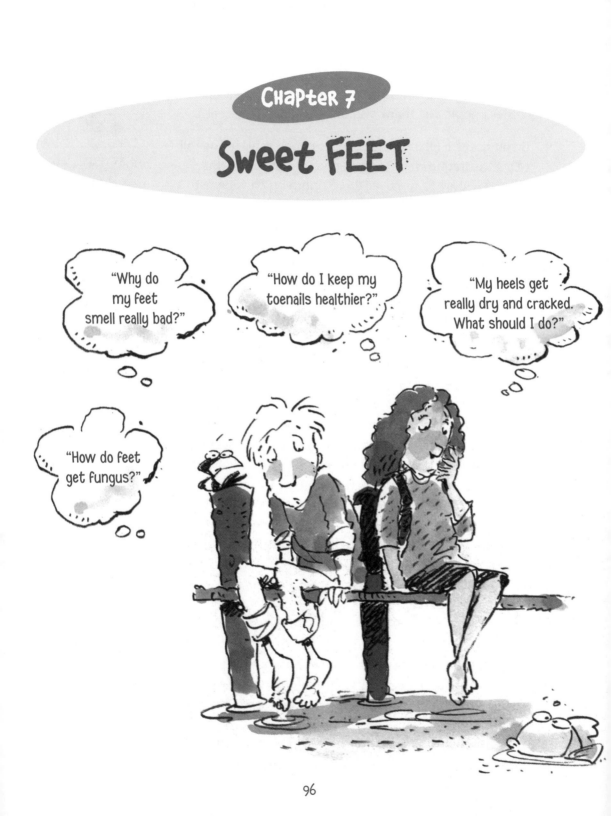

Take off your shoes and socks and inspect what's hiding underneath. How are your feet? Do you take good care of them? Are they clean and fresh? Or do they have funky-looking toenails, cracked skin, and a smell that could make a dog flinch? You've got some work to do if your feet fit that description. With a little effort, you can have a sweet pair of feet.

## FEET FACTS

Just before puberty, your hands and feet start to grow more quickly than other body parts. In fact, they're the first parts of your body to become adult sized. When you look down, you might notice that your feet are pretty big compared to other parts. The rest of your body will eventually catch up. Or perhaps you've noticed that your feet are smaller than everyone else's. You may be self-conscious or wonder if you look younger than your age.

Maybe you think your feet are ugly or funny looking. You may even try to hide them as much as possible. Keep in mind that everyone's feet have a unique shape and appearance. Some people have high arches in their feet, while some have flat feet. Some people's toes point inward; others point outward. Some feet are hairy, and some aren't.

You've probably never considered your feet to be a work of art. But Leonardo da Vinci—a genius of the fifteenth century—once called the human foot "a masterpiece of engineering and a work of art." Without your feet, you couldn't run, dance, kick a ball, climb the stairs, or ride your skateboard. Whenever you're tempted to criticize your feet for their size or shape, consider all they do for you. Your feet are quite a feat!

Fact!

There are 26 bones in each of your feet.

★

Look at the length of your forearm, from your elbow to your wrist. It's about the same length as one of your feet.

★

People usually have a dominant foot, which means they use it more often than the other one. Usually, the dominant foot is on the same side as the dominant hand. If someone kicks a ball toward you, which foot do you automatically use to stop the ball and kick it back? That's your dominant foot.

"My cousin took off her shoes one time, and they stunk really bad. Somebody said, 'Put your shoes back on! You're scaring the dogs!' She laughed and put them back on."
—Amanda, 12

"I have stinky feet. Every time I take my shoes off, I squint."
—Josh, 10

## Why Are Feet So Stinky?

Maybe you've been hiding your feet for another reason—because they stink. The most common complaint about our feet is that they smell. Well, there's a good reason for that.

Of the more than 2 million sweat glands in your body, most of them are found on the palms of your hands and soles of your feet. The sweat oozing from these glands doesn't have a smell, but the bacteria feeding on it do. And that's where foot odor starts. On average, your feet release about one half to one cup of sweat every day. The more sweat you produce, the more bacteria come to dine.

Think about what you wear on your feet. Most likely, you usually wear sneakers or other heavy shoes, plus socks. All the sweat on your feet can't evaporate when you've got shoes and socks on. This means a smelly mixture of sweat and bacteria brews inside each shoe all day long.

Bacteria love the warm, moist environment inside your shoes. To prevent stinky feet, try to keep your feet dry, dry, dry.

Here's a plan for keeping your feet drier and fresher:

✱ Wash them every morning with an antibacterial or a deodorant soap.

✱ Scrub your feet well with a washcloth to remove any dead skin. Make sure to wash between your toes.

✱ Dry your feet well after washing them. You can even use a hair dryer, if you want.

✱ If needed, use a foot product designed to cut down on sweat and odor. You can find lotions, creams, gels, powders, or sprays.

★ Avoid wearing the same shoes all the time. Every few days, put on a different pair of shoes and let the other pair air out. Set the shoes in a window or in front of a fan to freshen them, instead of tossing them in the back of a stuffy closet or under your bed.

★ If possible, wash your sneakers occasionally in the washing machine. Let them air dry. Don't put them in the dryer, or they might shrink.

★ Wear sandals, flip-flops, or clogs so your feet can "breathe."

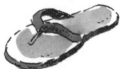

If you have an out-of-the-ordinary case of stinky feet, you can:

★ Apply an antiperspirant to your (clean) feet each morning and even at night before bed. Look for an ingredient called *aluminum chlorohydrate,* which will help keep your feet drier.

★ Sprinkle a mixture of one-part cornstarch to one-part baking soda in your socks to absorb sweat.

★ If you've really got a problem with perspiration and odor, you could try soaking your feet every day in a solution of black tea and cool water. Brew two tea bags in two cups of boiling water for 15 minutes. Add the tea to two quarts of cool water. Soak your feet for 20 to 30 minutes.

★ Change your socks several times a day, if necessary. Always choose cotton socks, because cotton "breathes" better than other fabrics.

★ If you continue to have problems with foot odor, talk to a doctor about prescribing a strong antiperspirant.

Fact!

The International Rotten Sneaker Stinkapalooza is held every year in Vermont. People from all parts of the world bring their stinky sneakers and compete for prizes.

"My feet are very stinky, and they sweat so much I feel like my shoe is a heater. I have to use foot odor powder because my feet stink up my shoes so bad."
—Caitlin, 10

## Fungus and Other Fun Stuff

If you play sports or are physically active, you may have had athlete's foot at some point. This fungal infection can show up on the skin of your feet or under your toenails. The term "athlete's foot" originally was created by an advertising company to help sell antifungal medication. Usually, people pick up this fungus in warm, moist places like showers in school locker rooms or gyms.

The symptoms of athlete's foot include itching and burning between the toes, a rash, and raw, flaking, cracking skin. (You may feel the urge to fling off your shoes and scratch like crazy!) You can easily treat athlete's foot with over-the-counter sprays or powders. It also helps to keep your feet dry.

To prevent getting the fungus in the first place, avoid walking around barefoot in public showers or pools. Instead, wear flip-flops to keep your feet off the moist floors or concrete.

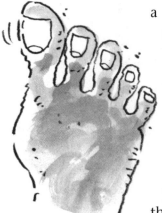

Another place fungus can grow is under your toenails. Nail fungus isn't pretty, but it can be treated. If you have a fungus, your toenails might be thick and yellow; they may also separate from the nail bed. You'll need to see a doctor who can diagnose the fungus and prescribe a treatment. Because toenails grow slowly (it may take a year to fully grow out a toenail), the treatment takes a long time.

Have you ever had an ingrown toenail? This is when the edge of the nail grows into the skin. Sometimes, ingrown toenails are caused by tight shoes or a fungus. No matter what the cause, ingrown toenails can be painful. You can ease the pain by soaking your sore toe in warm water. Be sure to keep the area clean to prevent infection.

To prevent ingrown toenails and the infections they may lead to, be sure to trim your nails every so often. Don't pick at them or tear them off—and definitely don't *bite* them. (Think of the germs!)

Trimming your toenails regularly will help them look neat and well cared for. To trim your toenails correctly, use a nail clipper and cut straight across. Don't trim them down too far, or you might hurt yourself. Push back the cuticles, just as you do with your fingernails (see pages 68–69 for more about that). Filing your toenails is optional. It may help you tame any rough edges.

Other foot problems include blisters, calluses, and corns. These are all minor problems, but they can irritate your feet in a big way.

Blisters usually are a result of your skin rubbing against your shoe. It's important to buy shoes that fit properly (read more about that on pages 102–104) to prevent blisters. If you get a blister, you may need to wear two pairs of socks for extra padding until it heals. You can wash the blister, put a disinfectant on it, and cover it with an adhesive bandage, as needed.

Calluses and corns form when your shoes rub against the bony areas of your feet. Calluses show up on the soles of your feet; corns are found on the tops of your toes. While the skin on your soles can be 10 times thicker than most of the skin on your body, a callous or corn can be 30 to 40 times thicker. You can treat corns and calluses by soaking your feet in warm water, drying them thoroughly, and then rubbing the corns and calluses with a pumice stone (you can find one in a drugstore). Apply a moisturizer to the thickened skin each day.

Maybe you've got a much simpler foot problem: dry skin. If the backs of your heels resemble a crocodile's skin, it's time to moisturize your feet. Start by soaking them in

## Fact!

If your big toe is longer than the one next to it, you have an advantage when it comes to sprinting. That big toe helps you accelerate more quickly.

✦

Abraham Lincoln had size 14 feet, which were huge compared to most men's feet in his day. He was flat-footed and pigeon-toed, which caused him to have painful corns. He often took off his boots when working in the White House; sometimes, he walked around in slippers because his feet hurt.

✦

When your foot "falls asleep," it's because you've been sitting or lying in a position that pressed on a nerve, which then stopped sending messages to your brain.

warm water to moisten the skin. Afterward, apply a generous helping of moisturizer and rub it in. If you really want to do the job right, put a layer of plastic wrap over each foot to seal in even more moisture. Then put on socks and stay this way overnight. Your feet will thank you in the morning.

## SHOE SAVVY

At your age, you might be interested in high heels, particularly if you're a girl. Have you ever seen someone wearing ridiculously high-heeled shoes that make her walk like she's tiptoeing around? She's on her way to foot trouble. Wearing shoes that are fashionable but hard on the feet can be a mistake.

High heels pitch your center of gravity forward; in response, you pull your shoulders back so you don't fall on your face. The result is that your back arches, which can lead to backaches. Experts also have found that high-heeled shoes cause a shortening of the tendon that runs up the back of the leg. To avoid these problems, stick with flat shoes or wear heels no higher than two inches.

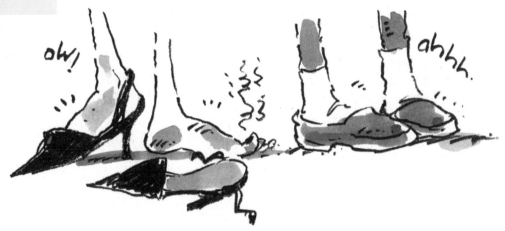

Shoes with pointed toes can cause problems, too. Look at your foot: Your toes don't come to a point. If they did, your big toe would be placed in the middle of your toes! Don't wear shoes with super-pointy toes, especially if you're going to be walking a lot. Instead, choose shoes that are more foot-friendly.

And how about those popular platform shoes? At least two young women have died from wearing platforms. Sound crazy? The high, chunky heels can be dangerous. A teacher died after falling off her shoes and suffering a skull fracture; a woman died in a car crash because her platform shoes got in the way of her reaching the brake. The chances of something like this happening to you are very rare, but platforms do have their pitfalls. Because these chunky heels are thicker than other high heels, people tend to wear them for longer periods of time, causing more back problems.

# ALL IN THE NAME OF FASHION

Centuries ago, Chinese women with tiny feet were considered feminine and beautiful. To make their feet as small as possible, wealthy Chinese women would tightly bind young girls' feet with bandages. The goal was to make the four smaller toes bend inward under the feet. After wearing the bandages for years, the girls' feet stopped growing. Sometimes, grown women had badly bent feet that were only four inches long. The women wore "lotus slippers," which looked like tiny, brightly colored baby booties, to draw attention to their tiny feet. Women with bound feet could walk only if someone helped them or by use of a cane. The practice of foot binding was stopped in 1902.

One of the best ways to treat your feet well is to buy the right shoes. Wearing comfortable, well-fitting shoes can save you lots of pain. You'll be more likely to avoid blisters, calluses, and corns if your shoes don't pinch or rub too hard against your skin.

"Why do I have small feet compared to other people? My mom has big feet and so does my dad, but I have 'Tiny Tim' feet."
—Reith, 9

As you probably know, shoes aren't cheap. They can be a big investment, so it's important to get the best pair for your money. Shop in stores that have knowledgeable sales people who can measure your feet and recommend shoes that will be comfortable and have the proper fit.

Here are some tips for smarter shoe shopping:

★ Shop in the afternoon when your feet are at their biggest size. (Feet swell as the day goes on.)

★ Try the shoes on with the socks you plan to wear with them, so you get a more accurate fit.

★ Don't buy shoes without trying them on first. At this point in your life, your feet are growing and changing quickly. Also, different brands of shoes may be sized differently.

★ It's possible you might have one foot that's larger than the other (lots of people do). Make sure the shoes you buy are sized to fit your largest foot.

★ The shoes should fit you snugly in the instep and at the heel. There should be at least a thumb's width of space between all your toes and the tip of the shoe.

★ Don't plan to "break shoes in." They should fit when you try them on.

★ Even though your feet might be growing like crazy, don't buy your shoes way too big or your feet will slide around in them.

★ Don't buy popular brands just because they're considered cool. They might be poorly made, expensive, and uncomfortable for you.

⭐ ⭐ ⭐

Feet can be a breeding ground for some strange beasts: bacteria, fungi, calluses, and corns. It's hard not to notice that feet can be one of the stinkiest parts of the body as well. But before you conclude that feet are disgusting or weird, remember that they help you get to the places you want to go. If you treat your feet right, there's no telling how far they might take you.

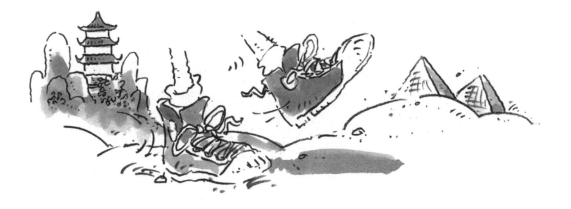

# A Final Word About Your UNIQUE PHYSIQUE

Throughout this book, you've learned how to take care of yourself from head to toe. Maybe you've discovered more about germs, bacteria, fungus, sweat, and stinky smells than you ever wanted to. There's one more important thing to know: Taking care of yourself isn't only "skin-deep." Here are 10 things you can do to take the best possible care of yourself from the inside out.

1. **MAKE THE BEST OF WHAT YOU'VE GOT.** We all have bodies of different shapes and sizes, and we mature at different rates. There's little point to sitting around worrying about whether you measure up to your friends or classmates. Instead, accept that your body is on its own timetable and that you're fine the way you are. You can help keep your body at its best by taking good care of what you've got.

2. **EAT THE RIGHT STUFF.** Are you a fast-food fan or junk-food junkie? Eating unhealthy foods once in a while is fine, but poor eating habits can catch up with you eventually. The grease from those French fries collect molecule by molecule in your arteries, leading to a possible heart attack or other health problems. So eat more fruits and vegetables, and fewer fries and shakes. You'll feel better, think better, and look better if you feed your body well.

3. **KNOW THAT "DIET" IS A DIRTY WORD.** Some of your friends, and possibly some adults in your life, are probably dieting right now. Keep in mind that skinny bodies aren't always *healthy* bodies. Because your body is growing and changing, it needs healthy foods, not a drastic cut in calories. The most important thing is to be strong and fit, and you can't be strong and fit without eating right.

4. **MOVE IT OR LOSE IT.** People can become out-of-shape "blobs" if they don't exercise. Many preteens and teens are couch potatoes; they sit inside watching TV, playing video games, or surfing the Internet. If you know more about the weekly TV lineup than you do about the walking routes in your neighborhood, it's time to get off the couch. Get your body in better shape by working out several times a week. You'll be proud of the muscles you can build.

5. **GET YOUR zzzzzzs.** When you're asleep, your body's growth hormones are wide awake and hard at work. In other words, you need sleep to grow! Many people your age are so busy they stay up late to finish everything, and then have to get up early for school. This leads to feeling tired, irritable, and unable to concentrate. Aim for about 8–10 hours of sleep per night. You'll feel healthier and more energetic if you get the rest you need.

6. **DON'T PICK UP THE HABIT.** Smoking stinks, it's addictive, it's expensive— and, eventually, it can kill you. Some people start smoking cigarettes in middle school to appear "cool." But there's nothing cool about what smoking can do to your health (or your appearance). Don't start a habit that's hard to break.

7. **BE SMART ABOUT DRUGS AND ALCOHOL.** These substances hurt your body and brain. They make it harder to stay healthy and fit, or think clearly. The truth is you've got enough to deal with as you grow into an adult. You'll handle the challenges of growing up more successfully if you avoid substances like these.

8. **BUST YOUR STRESS.** These days, you might be more stressed out as a result of changes in your life. Stress can cause symptoms like headaches, stomachaches, or diarrhea. To release stress, you can exercise and do deep breathing. Talk to someone about how you feel or any problems you may have. Finding a quiet place to relax and think peaceful thoughts can help, too.

9. **LEARN TO HANDLE YOUR EMOTIONS.** Puberty is an emotional time. You might feel happy one minute and depressed the next, or get mad at little things. These ups and downs are normal. Stay calm, think things through,

and find healthy ways to deal with your feelings. You can write in a journal or talk with a friend or an adult you trust. Most of all, understand that feelings are normal and you can handle them.

10. GET TO KNOW YOURSELF. You're starting to figure out who you are and to learn about your strengths and weaknesses. When you look at yourself, don't focus only on the negatives or put yourself down for making mistakes. Instead, think about the positives. What are your talents and interests? Think about what you'd like your life to be like and take steps to reach your goals. You'll feel better about yourself when you know who you are and what you want out of life.

# Where to Go for More Info

## BOOKS

*The Care & Keeping of You: The Body Book for Girls* by American Girl Library (Madison, WI: Pleasant Company Publications, 1998). This book is a guide to basic health and hygiene and offers a lot of information on a diverse selection of topics: hair, eyes, ears, mouth, skin, hands, acne, nutrition, exercise, puberty, periods, feet, sleep, and more.

*The Complete Idiot's Guide to Looking Great for Teens* by Ericka Lutz (Indianapolis, IN: Alpha Books, 2001). Written for boys and girls, this book offers advice on your health, fitness, and appearance. Learn how to stay fit and eat right, and get tips for taking care of your skin, finding your own personal style, and making smart choices about alcohol and drugs.

*What's Going on Down There? Answers to Questions Boys Find Hard to Ask* by Karen Gravelle with Nick and Chava Castro (New York: Walker & Co., 1998). This book answers many questions boys might have about puberty, from what it is and what it feels like, to what puberty is like for girls, to how to handle the sexual feelings you may be starting to experience.

*The What's Happening to My Body? Book for Boys* by Lynda Madaras (New York: Newmarket Press, 2000). Here you'll find a lot of information on your body and emotions, puberty, zits, facial hair, body odor, and more.

*The What's Happening to My Body? Book for Girls* by Lynda Madaras (New York: Newmarket Press, 2000). This book covers everything that you need to know about puberty and body changes. Find information on physical development, menstruation, emotions, and much more.

## WEB SITES

**American Academy of Dermatology Kids' Connection**
*www.aad.org/Kids/index.html*
This site provides you with information about your skin and potential skin conditions. Learn, for example, about skin diseases, the effects of the sun on your skin, and the benefits of sunscreen. You'll also find links to information about other skin issues, including acne.

**American Dental Association Kids' Corner**
*www.ada.org/public/topics/kids/index.html*
Find out why you need to visit the dentist and learn about cavities and other dental conditions. You can also find out the scoop on bad breath and learn how to maintain your bright smile.

**Discovery Health**

*yucky.kids.discovery.com*

Get the lowdown on ear wax, eye gunk, zits, dandruff, and more at this fun site that explores the mysterious, funny, and sometimes yucky ways your body works.

**KidsHealth**

*www.kidshealth.org*

This site has a huge variety of topics dealing with your health. The Kids' site offers information about your body and how to take care of it. There's a section on growing up that covers periods, puberty, braces and retainers, voice changes, and what's normal. The Teens' site has more in-depth information on acne, sexual development, and other issues that arise during puberty. Nutrition, fitness, and illness are covered at both sites.

**Powerful Bones. Powerful Girls.**

*www.cdc.gov/powerfulbones/index.html*

This colorful site offers fun facts and lots of information about your bones. Includes games, quizzes, recipes for calcium-filled treats, and sound advice on how to build stronger bones with calcium and weight-bearing exercises.

**TeenGrowth**

*www.teengrowth.com*

You'll find advice on dealing with emotions, family, and friends, as well as tons of great information on physical development, proper nutrition, and exercise. Find tips for avoiding unnecessary stress and other problems at home, in the classroom, and with friends.

# Bibliography

## BOOKS AND ARTICLES

Abner, Allison, and Linda Villarosa. *Finding Our Way: The Teen Girls' Survival Guide.* New York: HarperCollins Publishers, 1996.

Branzei, Sylvia. *Grossology.* Reading, MA: Addison-Wesley Publishing Company, 1996.

Branzei, Sylvia. *Grossology Begins at Home.* Reading, MA: Addison-Wesley Publishing Company, 1997.

Elfman, Eric. *Almanac of the Gross, Disgusting and Totally Repulsive.* New York: Random House, 1994.

Kerr, Daisy. *Keeping Clean: A Very Peculiar History.* New York: Franklin Watts, 1995.

Lawlor, Laurie. *Where Will This Shoe Take You? A Walk Through the History of Footwear.* New York: Walker and Company, 1996.

Leokum, Arkady. *Tell Me Why, #1.* New York: Grosset & Dunlap, 1986.

Madaras, Lynda. *The What's Happening to My Body? Book for Boys.* New York: Newmarket Press, 2000.

Masoff, Joy. *Oh Yuck! The Encyclopedia of Everything Nasty.* New York: Workman Publishing, 2000.

McCoy, Kathy, and Charles Wibbelsman. *The Teenage Body Book.* New York: The Berkley Publishing Group, 1992.

*Missouri Show-Me Your Smile: A Guide for Teaching Dental Health.* Jefferson City, MO: Missouri Department of Health, 1993.

Novick, Nelson. *Skin Care for Teens.* New York: Franklin Watts, 1988.

Pedersen, Stephanie. *Keep It Simple Series Guide to Beauty.* London: DK Publishing, Inc., 2001.

Porter, Alan. "Why Do We Have Apocrine and Sebaceous Glands?" *Journal of the Royal Society of Medicine* 94, 2001 (236–237).

Silverstein, Dr. Alvin and Virginia Silverstein. *The Story of Your Foot.* New York: G.P. Putnam's Sons, 1987.

Silverstein, Dr. Alvin, Virginia Silverstein, and Laura Silverstein Nunn. *Tooth Decay and Cavities.* New York: Franklin Watts, 2000.

Stewart, Alex. *Everyday History: Keeping Clean.* New York: Franklin Watts, 2000.

Walker, Richard. *The Children's Atlas of the Human Body.* Brookfield, CT: The Millbrook Press, 1994.

Walker, Ruth. "When in Halifax, Spare the Deodorant" *The Christian Science Monitor,* June 21, 2000.

Ward, Brian. *Dental Care.* London: Franklin Watts, 1986.

Weil, Andrew. "The Long and Short on Problem Nails" *Self Healing,* November 2001.

York-Goldman, Dianne and Mitchel Goldman. *Beauty Basics for Teens.* New York: Three Rivers Press, 2001.

# WEB SITES

Altruis Biomedical Network
*www.sweating.net, www.hairless.net, www.skin-information.com,* and *www.e-moisturizer.net*

American Academy of Dermatology
*www.aad.org*

American Academy of Pediatric Dentistry
*www.aapd.org*

American Dental Association
*www.ada.org*

American Podiatric Medical Association
*www.apma.org*

American Society for Microbiology
*www.washup.org*

Anderson, J., and L. Brown
"Nutrition and Dental Health" May 2001
*www.ext.colostate.edu/pubs/foodnut/09321.html*

Beautyworlds.com
*www.beautyworlds.com*

Case, Christine
"Handwashing," Jan. 8, 2002, Access Excellence @ the National Health Museum
*www.accessexcellence.org*

Center for Disease Control
*www.cdc.gov*

Discovery Health
*yucky.kids.discovery.com*

Go Ask Alice!
*www.goaskalice.columbia.edu*

KidsHealth
*www.kidshealth.org*

Medscape Health for Consumers
*www.health.medscape.com*

Museum of Menstruation and Women's Health
*www.mum.org*

News UC Davis
"New Invention Creates Odor-Free Socks, Infection-Fighting Scrubs," Oct. 3, 2000
*www.news.ucdavis.edu/newsreleases/10.00/news_odor-free_socks.html.*

Partnership for Food Safety Education
*www.fightbac.org*

Society of Chiropodists & Podiatrists
*www.feetforlife.org*

Useless Knowledge
*www.uselessknowledge.com*

Wolf, Buck
"The Smelly Foot Fest," Oct. 16, 2001
*www.abcnews.go.com/sections/us/WolfFiles/wolffiles106.html*

# Index

# About the Author

Marguerite Crump teaches health and physical education in the New Bloomfield R-III School District in New Bloomfield, Missouri. Crump has a master's degree in journalism from MU and one in physical education from Wichita State University. She has been a professional basketball player, a coach, a magazine editor, and a wellness coordinator. She lives in Columbia, Missouri, with her husband Joe. They have a feisty wiener dog named Sadie and a very patient cat named Molly.

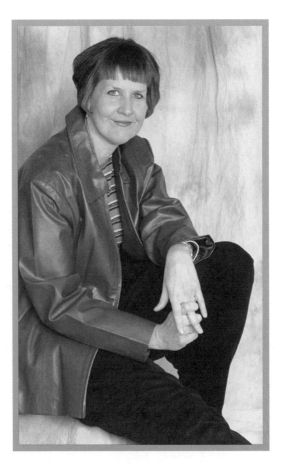

# Other Great Books from Free Spirit

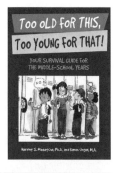

## Too Old for This, Too Young for That!
Your Survival Guide for the Middle-School Years
*by Harriet S. Mosatche, Ph.D., and Karen Unger, M.A.*
Finally there's a survival guide for the "tweens." Comprehensive, inter-active, friendly, and fun, meticulously researched and developmentally appropriate, this book addresses issues that matter to young people this age. Packed with quizzes, anecdotes, stories, surveys, and more, this is just what boys and girls need to make the most of middle school—and beyond. For ages 10–14.
*$14.95; 200 pp.; softcover; illus.; 7" x 9"*

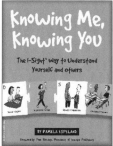

## Knowing Me, Knowing You
The I-Sight® Way to Understand Yourself and Others
*by Pamela Espeland*
Using the DiSC® dimensions of behavior (direct and active, interested and lively, steady and cooperative, concerned and correct), teens learn how their personal styles change from one situation to the next and explore ways to use this knowledge for more effective interactions with others. For ages 12 & up.
*$13.95; 128 pp.; softcover; illus.; 7" x 9"*

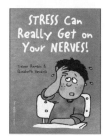

## Stress Can Really Get on Your NERVES!
*by Trevor Romain and Elizabeth Verdick*
More kids than ever feel worried, stressed out, and anxious every day. This book is a helping hand for those kids. Reassuring words, silly jokes, and light-hearted cartoons let them know they're not the only worry-warts on the planet—and they can learn to manage their stress. For ages 8–13.
*$9.95; 104 pp.; softcover; illus.; 5⅛" x 7"*

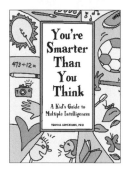

## You're Smarter Than You Think
A Kid's Guide to Multiple Intelligences
*by Thomas Armstrong, Ph.D.*
In clear, simple language, this book introduces the theory, explains the eight intelligences, and describes numerous ways to develop each one. Kids will learn how they can use all eight intelligences in school, expand their multiple intelligences at home, and draw on them to plan for the future. Resources point the way to books, software, games, and organizations that can help kids develop the eight intelligences. This timely, important book is recommended for all kids, their parents, and educators. For ages 8–12.
*$15.95; 192 pp.; softcover; illus.; 7" x 9"*

*To place an order or to request a free catalog of SELF–HELP FOR KIDS® and SELF–HELP FOR TEENS® materials, please write, call, email, or visit our Web site:*

**Free Spirit Publishing Inc.**
**217 Fifth Avenue North • Suite 200 • Minneapolis, MN 55401-1299**
**toll-free 800.735.7323 • local 612.338.2068 • fax 612.337.5050**
**help4kids@freespirit.com • www.freespirit.com**

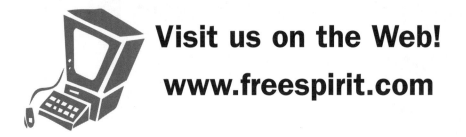

# Visit us on the Web!
# www.freespirit.com

Stop by anytime to find our Parents' Choice Approved catalog with fast, easy, secure 24-hour online ordering; "Ask Our Authors," where visitors ask questions—and authors give answers—on topics important to children, teens, parents, teachers, and others who care about kids; links to other Web sites we know and recommend; fun stuff for everyone, including quick tips and strategies from our books; and much more! Plus our site is completely searchable so you can find what you need in a hurry. Stop in and let us know what you think!

# Just point and click!

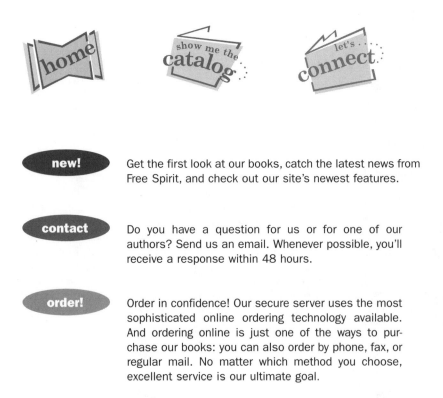

**new!** Get the first look at our books, catch the latest news from Free Spirit, and check out our site's newest features.

**contact** Do you have a question for us or for one of our authors? Send us an email. Whenever possible, you'll receive a response within 48 hours.

**order!** Order in confidence! Our secure server uses the most sophisticated online ordering technology available. And ordering online is just one of the ways to purchase our books: you can also order by phone, fax, or regular mail. No matter which method you choose, excellent service is our ultimate goal.

**1.800.735.7323 • fax 612.337.5050 • help4kids@freespirit.com**